Baby Name Book

30,000+ Meaningful, Timeless, and Unique Baby Names from Around the World to Help You Choose the Right Name for Your Baby

ISBN: 9798322338581

MANCUNIA PUBLISHING

Copyright © 2024 by Mancunia Publishing

All rights reserved. No part of this publication may be reproduced, distributed, or transmitted in any form or by any means, including photocopying, recording, or other electronic or mechanical methods, without the prior written permission of the publisher, except in the case of brief quotations embodied in critical reviews and certain other noncommercial uses permitted by copyright law.

TABLE OF CONTENTS

Introduction...8
Baby Names and Where They Come From................10
How to Name Your Baby..12
Name Trends 2024 (United States).........................15
Name Trends 2024 (United Kingdom)......................16
Name Trends 2024 (Canada)...................................17
Name Trends 2024 (Netherlands)............................19
Name Trends 2024 (Germany).................................20
Name Trends 2024 (Sweden)...................................21
American baby names and their meanings............22
British baby names and their meanings..................25
Canadian baby names and their meanings............28
Australian baby names and their meanings..........31
German baby names and their meanings...............34
French baby names and their meanings.................37
Italian baby names and their meanings.................40
Spanish baby names and their meanings...............43
Chinese baby names and their meanings..............46
Japanese baby names and their meanings............49
Indian baby names and their meanings.................52
Mexican baby names and their meanings..............55
Brazilian baby names and their meanings.............58
Russian baby names and their meanings...............61
Dutch baby names and their meanings..................64
Swedish baby names and their meanings..............67
Norwegian baby names and their meanings..........70
Danish baby names and their meanings................73
Finnish baby names and their meanings................76
Greek baby names and their meanings..................79
Turkish baby names and their meanings................82
Egyptian baby names and their meanings.............85
South African baby names and their meanings....88
Nigerian baby names and their meanings.............91
Kenyan baby names and their meanings................94
Ghanaian baby names and their meanings...........98

Ethiopian baby names and their meanings..........................101
Moroccan baby names and their meanings.......................104
Algerian baby names and their meanings.........................107
Tunisian baby names and their meanings..........................110
Libyan baby names and their meanings.............................113
Saudi Arabian baby names and their meanings.................116
Iranian baby names and their meanings.............................119
Iraqi baby names and their meanings..................................122
Israeli baby names and their meanings...............................126
Palestinian baby names and their meanings.....................129
Jordanian baby names and their meanings.......................132
Syrian baby names and their meanings..............................135
Lebanese baby names and their meanings.......................138
Kuwaiti baby names and their meanings............................141
Emirati baby names and their meanings............................144
Qatari baby names and their meanings..............................147
Omani baby names and their meanings.............................150
Bahraini baby names and their meanings..........................153
Pakistani baby names and their meanings........................157
Bangladeshi baby names and their meanings..................160
Sri Lankan baby names and their meanings.....................163
Nepali baby names and their meanings.............................166
Bhutanese baby names and their meanings....................169
Afghan baby names and their meanings...........................172
Kazakhstani baby names and their meanings..................175
Uzbekistani baby names and their meanings...................178
Tajikistani baby names and their meanings......................181
Kyrgyzstani baby names and their meanings...................184
Turkmenistani baby names and their meanings..............187
Mongolian baby names and their meanings.....................190
Vietnamese baby names and their meanings...................193
Thai baby names and their meanings.................................197
Malaysian baby names and their meanings......................200
Indonesian baby names and their meanings....................203
Filipino baby names and their meanings............................206
Singaporean baby names and their meanings.................210

Cambodian baby names and their meanings	213
Laotian baby names and their meanings	216
Bruneian baby names and their meanings	219
Taiwanese baby names and their meanings	222
Hong Kong baby names and their meanings	225
Macau baby names and their meanings	228
Tibetan baby names and their meanings	231
Maldivian baby names and their meanings	234
Mauritian baby names and their meanings	237
Seychellois baby names and their meanings	240
Malagasy baby names and their meanings	243
Mauritanian baby names and their meanings	246
Gambian baby names and their meanings	249
Senegalese baby names and their meanings	252
Guinean baby names and their meanings	255
Ivorian baby names and their meanings	258
Burkinabe baby names and their meanings	261
Ghanaian baby names and their meanings	264
Togolese baby names and their meanings	267
Beninese baby names and their meanings	270
Nigerian baby names and their meanings	273
Cameroonian baby names and their meanings	276
Gabonese baby names and their meanings	279
Equatorial Guinean baby names and their meanings	282
Congolese baby names and their meanings	285
Angolan baby names and their meanings	288
Namibian baby names and their meanings	291
Botswanan baby names and their meanings	294
Zimbabwean baby names and their meanings	297
Zambian baby names and their meanings	300
Malawian baby names and their meanings	303
Mozambican baby names and their meanings	306
Sudanese baby names and their meanings	309
Egyptian baby names and their meanings	312
Libyan baby names and their meanings	315
Algerian baby names and their meanings	318

Tunisian baby names and their meanings..................321
Christian Names..................324
Islamic Names..................327
Hindu Names..................328
Buddhist Names..................330
Jewish Names..................331
Sikh Names..................332
Millennial Baby Names..................333
1950s Baby Names..................335
1960s Baby Names..................336
1970s Baby Names..................337
1980s Baby Names..................339
1990s Baby Names..................340
Natural Baby Names..................343
Historical Figures Baby Names..................344
Ancient Roman Baby Names..................345
Ancient Greek Baby Names..................346
Celebrity Baby Names..................347
Pagan Baby Names..................349
Shakespeare Names..................353
Astrological Names..................356
Geographic Names..................360
Gender Neutral Names..................363
Ancient Irish Names..................365
Ancient Scottish Names..................371
Ancient English Names..................375
Ancient Latin Names..................377
Ancient Hebrew Names..................379
Ancient Arabic Names..................382
Ancient Eqyptian Names..................384
Royal Names..................386
Nautical Names..................388
Weather Names..................390
Literary Names..................392
Harry Potter™ Characters..................394
Native American Names..................396

Aboriginal Names..398
Maroi Names...399
Sami Names..401
Inuit Names...403
Hawiian Names...406
Military Names..409
Slavic Names...411
Saxon Names..414
Celtic Names...415
Ancient Welsh Names...417
Persian Names...419
Lucky Names..421
Food Based Names...422
Gem Names...423
Artist Names...426
Sports Stars Names..428
Saints Names...430
Political Leaders Names...432
Philosphers Names...434
Floral Names..437

Introduction

Welcome to The Baby Name Book, a treasure trove of inspiration for parents-to-be embarking on the exciting journey of choosing the perfect name for their little one. Within these pages, you'll find over 30,000 meaningful, timeless, and unique baby names sourced from diverse cultures and traditions around the world. Whether you're seeking a name that reflects your cultural heritage, resonates with personal significance, or simply captures your imagination, this book is your ultimate guide to finding the name that feels just right for your bundle of joy.

Choosing a name for your baby is one of the most significant decisions you'll make as a parent. It's a decision that carries with it the weight of shaping your child's identity and influencing how they perceive themselves and interact with the world. With so many names to choose from and countless factors to consider, the process can feel overwhelming. That's where The Baby Name Book comes in to simplify and enrich your search.

In the pages that follow, you'll embark on a journey across continents and cultures, exploring the rich tapestry of human naming traditions. From the classic elegance of European names to the lyrical beauty of names from Asia and Africa, each entry in this book is a window into the history, meaning, and cultural significance of names from around the globe.

But The Baby Name Book is more than just a list of names—it's a celebration of diversity, heritage, and the boundless creativity of human expression.

In addition to providing a vast array of name options, The Baby Name Book also offers practical guidance and insights to help you navigate the naming process with confidence. From tips for narrowing down your options to considerations for honoring family traditions and cultural heritage, this book is your trusted companion every step of the way.

As you embark on this exciting journey of naming your baby, remember that the perfect name is one that resonates with your heart and soul, evoking a sense of joy, meaning, and connection. Whether you're seeking a name steeped in tradition or one that breaks new ground, The Baby Name Book is here to inspire and empower you as you welcome your little one into the world.

So dive in, explore, and discover the name that will be a cherished part of your family's story for generations to come. The adventure begins here in The Baby Name Book—a celebration of the power and beauty of names, and the boundless love that awaits your precious bundle of joy.

Baby Names and Where They Come From

In the vast and diverse landscape of human culture, names serve as more than mere labels—they are a reflection of history, tradition, and identity. From the ancient civilizations of Mesopotamia to the contemporary melting pot of global society, the origins of baby names are as varied and fascinating as the cultures that inspire them. In this chapter, we'll embark on a journey through time and space, exploring the rich tapestry of naming traditions from around the world.

Ancient Origins:

The practice of naming children is as old as human civilization itself. In ancient societies, names often carried deep significance, reflecting the hopes, beliefs, and values of parents and communities. In Mesopotamia, one of the cradles of civilization, names like Gilgamesh and Ishtar harkened back to the myths and deities of Sumerian and Babylonian culture. Meanwhile, in ancient Egypt, names such as Ramses and Cleopatra were imbued with royal lineage and divine authority, symbolizing power and prestige.

European Elegance:

As civilization spread across Europe, so too did a rich tapestry of naming traditions. In medieval times, names like William and Elizabeth were popular among the English nobility, while names like Giovanni and Maria held sway in Italy. In Scandinavia, names like Erik and Ingrid drew inspiration from Norse mythology, invoking the bravery of legendary warriors and the beauty of nature. From the romantic allure of French names to the timeless charm of Germanic names, Europe has been a wellspring of inspiration for parents seeking names that are both classic and sophisticated.

Cultural Kaleidoscope:

In the global mosaic of culture, names serve as a vibrant expression of diversity and heritage. From the rhythmic cadence of African names to the lyrical beauty of Asian names, every corner of the globe boasts its own unique naming traditions. In Africa, names like Kwame and Nala often carry deep symbolic meanings, reflecting concepts like strength, wisdom, and spirituality. In Asia, names like Aarav and Mei evoke images of natural beauty and cultural pride, while in the Americas, names like Maya and Diego celebrate indigenous heritage and resilience.

Modern Trends:

In today's interconnected world, naming trends are constantly evolving, shaped by factors like pop culture, celebrity influence, and technological innovation. From the rise of gender-neutral names like Taylor and Jordan to the resurgence of vintage names like Evelyn and Henry, parents have more options than ever before. Meanwhile, the digital age has given rise to a new frontier of naming possibilities, with names like Alexa and Elon reflecting the influence of technology and entrepreneurship.

How to Name Your Baby

Naming your baby is a deeply personal and meaningful experience—a decision that will shape their identity for a lifetime. With so many options to consider, from traditional family names to modern innovations, the task can seem daunting. In this chapter, we'll explore some practical tips and heartfelt considerations to help guide you through the process of choosing the perfect name for your little one.

1. Start Early:

While it's tempting to leave naming until after your baby arrives, starting the brainstorming process early can alleviate stress and give you ample time to explore your options. Begin compiling a list of potential names as soon as you learn you're expecting, allowing plenty of time for research and reflection.

2. Consider Your Values and Beliefs:

Names often carry deep significance, reflecting the values, beliefs, and cultural heritage of parents and families. Take some time to consider what qualities you hope to instill in your child and how you want their name to reflect those ideals. Whether you're drawn to traditional names with deep roots or modern names with contemporary flair, let your values be your guide.

3. Seek Inspiration:

Drawing inspiration from a variety of sources can help spark creativity and open up new possibilities. Explore literature, mythology, history, and nature for inspiration, as well as your own family tree for meaningful family names and traditions. Websites, books, and baby name apps can also be valuable resources for discovering new names and learning their meanings.

4. Consider Sound and Spelling:

When choosing a name, consider how it sounds when spoken aloud and how it pairs with your last name. Pay attention to the rhythm, flow, and pronunciation of the name, as well as potential nicknames or abbreviations. Similarly, consider the spelling of the name and whether it might lead to confusion or mispronunciation.

5. Think Long-Term:

While it's important to choose a name that feels right in the moment, it's also wise to think long-term and consider how the name will age with your child. Avoid trendy or faddish names that may feel dated in a few years, opting instead for names that are timeless and enduring.

6. Get Feedback:

Once you've narrowed down your list of potential names, don't hesitate to seek feedback from trusted friends and family members. Keep in mind, however, that ultimately the decision is yours and your partner's, so choose a name that resonates with you both.

7. Trust Your Instincts:

In the end, the most important thing is to choose a name that feels right for you and your family. Trust your instincts and go with the name that fills you with joy and excitement. Remember, your baby's name is a reflection of your love and hopes for their future, so choose with confidence and cherish the journey of naming your little one.

Name Trends 2024 (United States)

Girls:

Emma, Olivia, Ava, Isabella, Sophia, Mia, Amelia, Harper, Evelyn, Abigail, Charlotte, Emily, Elizabeth, Avery, Sofia, Ella, Madison, Scarlett, Grace, Lily, Chloe, Zoey, Layla, Natalie, Hannah, Victoria, Aria, Aurora, Stella, Penelope, Riley, Nora, Zoey, Ellie, Lily, Maya, Aubrey, Adeline, Hannah, Lucy, Madelyn, Eleanor, Hazel, Lillian, Skylar, Claire, Isabelle, Addison, Brooklyn, Paisley, Savannah, Naomi, Elena, Caroline, Kennedy, Genesis, Autumn, Emilia, Cora, Reagan, Serenity, Piper, Ariana, Kaylee, Julia, Valentina, Katherine, Faith, Sadie, Sydney, Alexa, Ximena, Hailey, Bella, Vivian, Eliana, Clara, Jasmine, Delilah, Jade, Ellie, Sophie, Zoe, Peyton, Mackenzie, Brielle, Taylor, Ruby, Lauren, Alice, Hadley, Violet, Aaliyah, Gabriella, Arianna, Kayla, Annabelle, Alyssa, Kinsley, Isla

Boys:

Liam, Noah, Oliver, Elijah, William, James, Benjamin, Lucas, Henry, Alexander, Mason, Michael, Ethan, Daniel, Logan, Matthew, Jackson, David, Joseph, Samuel, Sebastian, Carter, Jayden, Wyatt, John, Owen, Gabriel, Dylan, Luke, Isaac, Christopher, Joshua, Andrew, Julian, Mateo, Ryan, Jack, Nathan, Caleb, Levi, Evan, Aaron, Cameron, Christian, Colton, Landon, Nicholas, Connor, Jeremiah, Josiah, Adrian, Leo, Hudson, Robert, Angel, Brayden, Gavin, Dominic, Austin, Jordan, Lincoln, Adam, Ian, Elias, Thomas, Xavier, Zachary, Nolan, Max, Chase, Cole, Brody, Grayson, Oscar, Tyler, Parker, Ryder, Diego, Luis, Wesley, Kai, Jace, Finn, Emmett, Harrison, Roman, Bennett, George, Victor, Miles

Name Trends 2024 (United Kingdom)

Girls:

Olivia, Amelia, Isla, Ava, Emily, Mia, Isabella, Sophia, Ella, Grace, Lily, Freya, Charlotte, Evie, Sophie, Jessica, Daisy, Alice, Willow, Ivy, Harper, Rosie, Matilda, Elsie, Ruby, Florence, Esme, Sienna, Phoebe, Evelyn, Chloe, Scarlett, Eliza, Millie, Poppy, Erin, Maisie, Eleanor, Hannah, Lucy, Georgia, Aria, Bella, Emilia, Molly, Abigail, Thea, Lottie, Penelope, Arabella, Aurora, Imogen, Zara, Clara, Harriet, Anna, Darcie, Heidi, Martha, Amber, Robyn, Gracie, Victoria, Jasmine, Lara, Nancy, Beatrice, Lydia, Violet, Bonnie, Hallie, Delilah, Frankie, Iris, Maddison, Lola, Bethany, Summer, Ayla

Boys:

Oliver, George, Harry, Noah, Jack, Leo, Arthur, Oscar, Charlie, Muhammad, Henry, Freddie, Alfie, Archie, Joshua, Ethan, Thomas, James, William, Max, Isaac, Alexander, Samuel, Daniel, Edward, Joseph, Sebastian, Finn, Theo, Teddy, Hugo, Jacob, Dylan, Albie, Tommy, Louie, Bobby, Jesse, Michael, Luca, Ronnie, Reuben, Elijah, Jake, Frankie, Jaxon, Sonny, Albert, Ollie, Gabriel, Eli, Rory, Reggie, Toby, Jenson, Caleb, Billy, Elliott, Jackson, Harley, Jude, Carter, Harvey, Seth, Luke, Stanley, Dexter

Name Trends 2024 (Canada)

Girls:

Olivia, Emma, Charlotte, Sophia, Ava, Mia, Amelia, Harper, Emily, Abigail, Isabella, Ella, Chloe, Lily, Aria, Avery, Grace, Zoey, Hannah, Victoria, Ellie, Nora, Scarlett, Maya, Addison, Aurora, Zoe, Emilia, Leah, Samantha, Lucy, Stella, Sarah, Claire, Eva, Penelope, Isla, Audrey, Layla, Anna, Mila, Ruby, Sadie, Nova, Brooklyn, Aaliyah, Gabriella, Peyton, Violet, Skylar, Hailey, Elizabeth, Willow, Alexis, Natalie, Savannah, Ariana, Eleanor, Bella, Mackenzie, Taylor, Arianna, Quinn, Clara, Alice, Sofia, Isabelle, Addison, Caroline, Madelyn, Paisley, Melanie, Arielle, Annabelle, Jasmine, Faith, Lila, Sydney, Kennedy.

Boys:

Liam, Noah, Jackson, Lucas, Oliver, Ethan, Benjamin, William, Henry, James, Alexander, Elijah, Mason, Logan, Carter, Jacob, Samuel, Owen, Jack, Leo, Wyatt, Aiden, Sebastian, Matthew, Gabriel, Lincoln, Nathan, Isaac, Thomas, Evan, Daniel, Connor, Theodore, Hudson, Caleb, Joshua, Hunter, Levi, Julian, Cooper, Jaxon, Nicholas, Dylan, Charlie, Ryder, Zachary, Gavin, Dominic, Maxwell, Adam, Eli, Tyler, Austin, Cameron, Ryan, Nolan, Cole, Lucas, Chase, Isaiah, Parker.

Name Trends 2024 (Australia)

Girls:

Charlotte, Olivia, Amelia, Mia, Ava, Isla, Grace, Harper, Sophie, Ella, Chloe, Emily, Ruby, Lily, Isabella, Sienna, Matilda, Zoe, Evelyn, Ivy, Scarlett, Willow, Lucy, Eva, Evie, Aria, Ellie, Hannah, Madison, Layla, Zara, Georgia, Jasmine, Chelsea, Lara, Abigail, Alice, Penelope, Violet, Stella, Molly, Savannah, Elsie, Rosie, Aurora, Annabelle, Claire, Phoebe, Hazel, Indie, Sofia, Addison, Alexis, Audrey, Eleanor, Eliza, Madeline, Alyssa, Mila, Charlie, Esme, Holly, Imogen, Jessica, Mackenzie, Milla, Piper, Poppy, Tahlia, Ayla, Eden, Elena, Emma, Heidi, Jade, Keira, Layla, Leila, Lola.

Boys:

Oliver, Noah, Jack, William, Leo, James, Thomas, Ethan, Lucas, Henry, Charlie, Mason, Liam, Alexander, Samuel, Benjamin, Lachlan, Max, Harrison, Oscar, Archie, Joshua, Isaac, Xavier, Hunter, Levi, Cooper, Theodore, Finn, Elijah, Jacob, Jackson, Harry, Riley, Luca, Harvey, Dylan, Connor, Tyler, Angus, George, Zachary, Carter, Jordan, Sebastian, Aiden, Patrick, Edward, Ryan, Jayden, Blake, Eli, Nate, Alex, Caleb, Daniel, Jaxon, Toby, Flynn, Lincoln, Louis, Mitchell, Kai, Matthew, Hamish, Hugo, Luke, Marcus, Archer, Bailey, Christopher, David, Dominic, Elliott, Felix, Jake, Jasper, Jesse, John, Jude, Nathan, Owen, Phoenix, Spencer, Adam, Ashton, Braxton, Brody.

Name Trends 2024 (Netherlands)

Girls:

Emma, Tess, Sophie, Julia, Mila, Anna, Sara, Zoe, Evi, Nora, Liv, Noa, Eva, Saar, Lotte, Lisa, Fleur, Lynn, Olivia, Nova, Isa, Lieke, Emily, Sarah, Zoë.

Boys:

Daan, Sem, Noah, Lucas, Finn, Liam, Levi, Milan, Luuk, Bram, Jesse, Mees, Thomas, Adam, Thijs, Lars, Max, Ruben, Noud, Sam, James, Julian.

Name Trends 2024 (Germany)

Girls:

Emma, Mia, Emilia, Hannah, Sophia, Sofia, Lina, Mila, Marie, Ella, Leni, Amelie, Clara, Leonie, Anna, Lena, Johanna, Lea, Nele, Lara, Maria, Sophie, Laura, Lotta, Amalia, Greta, Elisa, Lia, Mathilda, Maja, Charlotte, Marlene, Pauline, Emely, Frieda, Frida, Jana, Antonia, Pia, Melina, Isabella, Helena, Emily, Maya, Zoe, Victoria, Julia, Jule, Ronja, Luise, Romy, Klara, Fiona, Mara, Katharina, Helene, Lisa, Miriam, Selina, Isabel, Leona, Mira, Hanna.

Boys:

Ben, Paul, Finn, Leon, Luis, Jonas, Noah, Felix, Max, Elias, Luca, Henry, Oskar, Theo, Anton, Jakob, Emil, Lenn, Arthur, Matteo, Samuel, Liam, Levi, Leo, Friedrich, Niklas, Vincent, Finn, Alexander, Adam, Carl, Tom, Moritz, Jannik, Julian, David, Bruno, Nils, Jonas, Ben

Name Trends 2024 (Sweden)

Girls:

Alice, Lilly, Astrid, Maja, Elsa, Alva, Olivia, Agnes, Vera, Ebba, Selma, Elvira, Wilma, Alma, Ellen, Nova, Signe, Filippa, Saga, Tilda, Frida, Isabella, Iris, Linnea, Lovisa, Emma, Stella, Hilda, Nellie, Ingrid, Hedvig, Julia, Lykke, Meja, Melina, Sigrid, Juni, Emilia, Tuva, Leia, Freja, Moa, Rut, Cornelia, Smilla, Elise, Tindra, Celine, Lova, Amanda, Jasmine, Ronja, Alba, Johanna, Ester, Melinda, Enya, Thea, Sally, Inez, Tilde

Boys:

Lucas, Liam, William, Oscar, Noah, Elias, Hugo, Adam, Alexander, Leo, Charlie, Oliver, Axel, Elliot, Albin, Ludvig, Theo, Gabriel, Adrian, Isak, August, Gustav, Anton, Carl, Elton, Melvin, Alfred, Vincent, Milton, Ville, Harry, Max, Noa, Sixten, Wilmer, Jonathan, Otto, Malte, Henry, Lo, Algot, Arvid, Ebbe, John, Edward, Elliott

American baby names and their meanings

1. Abigail - Father's joy
2. Addison - Son of Adam
3. Alexander - Defender of mankind
4. Amelia - Industrious
5. Andrew - Manly, brave
6. Anna - Grace
7. Anthony - Priceless one
8. Ava - Bird
9. Benjamin - Son of the right hand
10. Brandon - From the broom hill
11. Charlotte - Free woman
12. Christopher - Christ-bearer
13. David - Beloved
14. Dylan - Son of the sea
15. Elizabeth - God is my oath
16. Emily - Industrious
17. Ethan - Firm, enduring
18. Grace - Grace of God
19. Hannah - Grace
20. Hunter - One who hunts
21. Isabella - God is my oath
22. Jack - God is gracious
23. Jacob - Supplanter
24. James - Supplanter
25. John - God is gracious
26. Joshua - God is salvation
27. Kayla - Pure
28. Liam - Strong-willed warrior
29. Madison - Son of Maud
30. Matthew - Gift of God
31. Mia - Mine
32. Michael - Who is like God?
33. Noah - Rest, comfort
34. Olivia - Olive tree

35. Sophia - Wisdom
36. William - Resolute protector
37. Zachary - God has remembered
38. Abner - Father of light
39. Bella - Beautiful
40. Caleb - Faithful
41. Daniel - God is my judge
42. Emma - Whole or universal
43. Faith - Trust, belief
44. Gabriel - God is my strength
45. Harper - Harp player
46. Isaac - He will laugh
47. Jessica - God beholds
48. Kaden - Companion
49. Layla - Night
50. Mason - Worker in stone
51. Natalie - Born on Christmas Day
52. Owen - Young warrior
53. Peyton - Fighting man's estate
54. Quinn - Wisdom, reason
55. Ryan - Little king
56. Sarah - Princess
57. Tyler - Tile maker
58. Victoria - Victory
59. Wyatt - Brave in war
60. Xavier - New house
61. Yasmine - Jasmine flower
62. Zoe - Life
63. Aaron - Exalted, strong
64. Brooke - Small stream
65. Carter - Transporter of goods by cart
66. Destiny - Fate
67. Elijah - My God is Yahweh
68. Fiona - Fair, white, beautiful
69. George - Farmer
70. Hazel - The hazelnut tree

71. Ivy - Faithfulness
72. Justin - Just, fair
73. Kennedy - Ugly head
74. Logan - Small hollow
75. Maya - Water
76. Nathan - He gave
77. Opal - Jewel
78. Penelope - Weaver
79. Riley - Rye clearing
80. Savannah - Flat tropical grassland
81. Tristan - Tumult, outcry
82. Ursula - Little bear
83. Violet - Purple/blue flower
84. Wesley - Western meadow
85. Xander - Defender of the people
86. Yasmin - Jasmine flower
87. Zachariah - God has remembered
88. Aurora - Dawn
89. Bentley - Meadow with coarse grass
90. Caroline - Free woman
91. Donovan - Dark
92. Evangeline - Bearer of good news
93. Finn - Fair
94. Genesis - Origin, creation
95. Hudson - Son of Hudd
96. Isla - Island
97. Jasper - Bringer of treasure
98. Kinsley - King's meadow
99. Leo - Lion
100. Molly - Star of the sea

British baby names and their meanings

1. Amelia - Industrious, striving
2. Olivia - Olive tree
3. Emily - Rival, eager
4. Ava - Bird
5. Isla - Island
6. Jessica - God beholds
7. Poppy - Red flower
8. Isabella - God is my oath
9. Sophie - Wisdom
10. Mia - Mine
11. Ruby - Red gemstone
12. Lily - Pure, passion
13. Grace - God's favor
14. Evie - Life
15. Charlotte - Free man
16. Scarlett - Red
17. Chloe - Blooming
18. Matilda - Battle-mighty
19. Lucy - Light
20. Ellie - Bright shining one
21. Freya - Noble woman
22. Alice - Noble, kind
23. Florence - Blossoming, flourishing
24. Sienna - Orange-red
25. Daisy - Day's eye, also a flower
26. Phoebe - Bright, pure
27. Millie - Gentle strength
28. Rosie - Rose
29. Imogen - Innocent, blameless
30. Lola - Sorrow
31. Harriet - Estate ruler
32. Eva - Life
33. Erin - Ireland
34. Martha - The lady

35. Holly - Plant with red berries
36. Molly - Star of the sea
37. Megan - Pearl
38. Maisie - Pearl
39. Bethany - House of figs
40. Jade - Green gemstone
41. Amber - Fossilized tree resin
42. Amelie - Hardworking
43. Harlow - Army hill
44. Heidi - Noble, kind
45. Georgia - Farmer
46. Summer - Season
47. Jasmine - Flower
48. Bella - Beautiful
49. Skye - Referring to the Isle of Skye in Scotland
50. Willow - Slender, graceful
51. Felix - Happy, fortunate
52. Oscar - Divine spear
53. Oliver - Olive tree
54. Jack - God is gracious
55. Harry - Army ruler
56. George - Farmer
57. Noah - Rest, comfort
58. Leo - Lion
59. Charlie - Free man
60. Jacob - Supplanter
61. Alfie - Wise counselor
62. Freddie - Peaceful ruler
63. Max - Greatest
64. Henry - Estate ruler
65. Joshua - God is salvation
66. Archie - Truly brave
67. Ethan - Strong, firm
68. Thomas - Twin
69. James - Supplanter
70. William - Resolute protector

71. Alexander - Defender of mankind
72. Archie - Truly brave
73. Benjamin - Son of the right hand
74. Daniel - God is my judge
75. Samuel - God has heard
76. Joseph - God will increase
77. Lucas - Light
78. Adam - Man, earth
79. Dylan - Son of the sea
80. Zac - God remembers
81. Riley - Rye clearing
82. Teddy - Wealthy protector
83. Toby - God is good
84. Ryan - Little king
85. Lewis - Famous warrior
86. Elijah - Yahweh is God
87. Finn - Fair
88. Elliot - Jehovah is God
89. Jayden - Thankful
90. Cameron - Crooked nose
91. Isaac - He will laugh
92. Mason - Stoneworker
93. Alex - Defender of mankind
94. Logan - Small hollow
95. Aaron - High mountain
96. Harrison - Son of Harry
97. Sebastian - Venerable, revered
98. Aiden - Little and fiery
99. Liam - Strong-willed warrior
100. Nathan - He gave

Canadian baby names and their meanings

1. Abigail - Father's joy
2. Alexander - Defender of mankind
3. Amelia - Industrious, striving
4. Andrew - Manly, brave
5. Ava - Life
6. Benjamin - Son of the right hand
7. Charlotte - Free woman
8. Daniel - God is my judge
9. Emily - Industrious, striving
10. Ethan - Firm, strong
11. Isabella - Devoted to God
12. Jacob - Supplanter
13. Liam - Resolute protector
14. Madison - Son of Maud
15. Noah - Rest, peace
16. Olivia - Olive tree
17. Sophia - Wisdom
18. William - Resolute protector
19. Zoe - Life
20. Jack - God is gracious
21. Aiden - Little fire
22. Harper - Harp player
23. Lucas - Light
24. Logan - Small hollow
25. Mason - Stoneworker
26. Emma - Universal
27. Grace - Goodness, generosity
28. Hannah - Grace of God
29. Jackson - Son of Jack
30. Lily - Purity, beauty
31. Michael - Who is like God?
32. Nathan - He gave
33. Owen - Young warrior
34. Penelope - Weaver

35. Quinn - Wise, intelligent
36. Riley - Courageous
37. Samuel - God has heard
38. Taylor - Tailor
39. Victoria - Victory
40. Wyatt - Brave in war
41. Xavier - The new house
42. Zachary - God has remembered
43. Audrey - Noble strength
44. Brooke - Small stream
45. Carter - Transporter of goods by cart
46. Dylan - Son of the sea
47. Evelyn - Desired
48. Finn - Fair
49. Gabriella - God is my strength
50. Harper - Harp player
51. Isaac - Laughter
52. Jasmine - Gift from God
53. Kayla - Pure
54. Leo - Lion
55. Mia - Mine
56. Natalie - Born on Christmas day
57. Oscar - Friend of deer
58. Paige - Young servant
59. Ryan - Little king
60. Scarlett - Red
61. Tristan - Tumult, outcry
62. Ursula - Little bear
63. Violet - Purple/blue flower
64. Wayne - Wagon maker
65. Xavier - Bright, splendid
66. Yvonne - Yew wood
67. Zachary - God remembered
68. Aaron - Exalted, strong
69. Bella - Beautiful
70. Caleb - Faithful, bold

71. Daisy - Day's eye
72. Ethan - Strong, firm
73. Faith - Trust, belief
74. George - Farmer
75. Hazel - The hazel tree
76. Ian - God is gracious
77. Julia - Youthful
78. Kyle - Narrow strait
79. Lauren - Laurel tree
80. Matthew - Gift of God
81. Nicole - Victory of the people
82. Oliver - Olive tree
83. Peyton - Fighting man's estate
84. Quinn - Wisdom, reason
85. Rose - Rose flower
86. Steven - Crown, garland
87. Tiffany - Manifestation of God
88. Ulysses - Wounded in the thigh
89. Vanessa - Butterfly
90. Wendy - Friend or blessed ring
91. Xavier - New house
92. Yolanda - Violet flower
93. Zachary - God has remembered
94. Ariel - Lion of God
95. Bentley - Meadow with coarse grass
96. Claire - Bright, clear
97. Derek - Ruler of the people
98. Elise - God is my oath
99. Frederick - Peaceful ruler
100. Gloria - Glory

Australian baby names and their meanings

1. Abigail - Source of Joy
2. Adelaide - Noble, Kind
3. Amelia - Industrious, Admiring
4. Ava - Like a Bird
5. Bella - Beautiful, God is my Oath
6. Charlotte - Free Woman
7. Chloe - Blooming, Fertility
8. Daisy - Day's Eye, Fresh, Bright
9. Ella - Beautiful Fairy Woman
10. Emily - Industrious, Striving
11. Freya - Lady, Noble Woman
12. Grace - God's Favor, Charm
13. Hannah - Grace of God
14. Isabella - God is my Oath
15. Jasmine - Gift from God, Flower
16. Kaitlyn - Pure
17. Lily - Purity, Beauty
18. Maddison - Son of the Mighty Warrior
19. Natalie - Born on Christmas Day
20. Olivia - Olive Tree
21. Poppy - Red Flower
22. Ruby - Red Gemstone
23. Scarlett - Bright Red
24. Sophia - Wisdom
25. Zoe - Life
26. Aaron - High Mountain, Enlightened
27. Benjamin - Son of the Right Hand
28. Charlie - Free Man
29. Daniel - God is my Judge
30. Ethan - Strong, Firm
31. Finn - Fair, White
32. George - Farmer
33. Harry - Home Ruler
34. Isaac - He will Laugh

35. Jack - God is Gracious
36. Kai - Sea
37. Liam - Strong-willed Warrior
38. Mason - Stoneworker
39. Noah - Rest, Comfort
40. Oliver - Olive Tree
41. Patrick - Nobleman
42. Quinn - Wise, Intelligent
43. Ryan - Little King
44. Samuel - Asked of God
45. Thomas - Twin
46. William - Resolute Protector
47. Xavier - Bright, Splendid
48. Zachary - God Remembers
49. Amber - Fossilized Tree Resin or Color Orange/Red
50. Bethany - House of Figs
51. Caitlin - Pure
52. Delilah - Delicate
53. Ebony - Dark Black-Wood
54. Faith - Trust, Belief
55. Gemma - Jewel
56. Harper - Harp Player
57. Ivy - Faithfulness
58. Jade - Green Gemstone
59. Kayla - Pure
60. Leah - Weary
61. Mia - Mine
62. Naomi - Pleasantness
63. Opal - Jewel, Gem
64. Paige - Assistant, Helper
65. Quinn - Wisdom, Reason
66. Rachel - Ewe, Sheep
67. Savannah - Treeless Plain
68. Taylor - Tailor
69. Ursula - Little Bear
70. Violet - Purple/Blue Flower

71. Willow - Slender, Graceful
72. Xanthe - Golden, Yellow
73. Yvonne - Yew, Archer
74. Zara - Blooming Flower
75. Adam - Man, To Make
76. Blake - Dark, Fair
77. Cooper - Barrel Maker
78. Dexter - Dyer, Right-Handed
79. Elijah - My God is Yahweh
80. Felix - Happy, Fortunate
81. Gavin - White Hawk
82. Hunter - One Who Hunts
83. Ivan - God is Gracious
84. Jasper - Treasurer
85. Kaden - Fighter
86. Levi - Joined, Attached
87. Max - Greatest
88. Nolan - Champion
89. Oscar - Friend of Deer
90. Preston - Priest's Town
91. Quentin - Fifth
92. Riley - Rye Clearing
93. Sebastian - Venerable, Revered
94. Tristan - Tumult, Outcry
95. Uriah - God is my Light
96. Victor - Winner, Conqueror
97. Wyatt - Brave in War
98. Xavier - The New House
99. York - Yew Tree Estate
100. Zane - God is Gracious

German baby names and their meanings

1. Ada – Noble, kind
2. Adalbert – Noble and bright
3. Adelina – Noble, kind
4. Alaric – Ruler of all
5. Albert – Noble, bright
6. Aldo – Old, wise
7. Amalia – Work of the Lord
8. Ansel – God's protection
9. Aric – Ruler of all
10. Arnold – Eagle power
11. August – Majestic
12. Axel – Father of peace
13. Beatrice – Bringer of joy
14. Bernd – Brave as a bear
15. Bernhard – Brave as a bear
16. Bruno – Brown
17. Carl – Free man
18. Caroline – Free woman
19. Clara – Clear, bright
20. Conrad – Bold counsel
21. Dagmar – Glorious day
22. Dietrich – Ruler of the people
23. Dorothea – Gift of God
24. Eckhart – Point of a sword
25. Edel – Noble
26. Elke – Noble, kind
27. Emil – Rival
28. Erich – Eternal ruler
29. Ernst – Serious, resolute
30. Eva – Life
31. Felix – Happy, fortunate
32. Ferdinand – Brave journey
33. Franz – Free man
34. Friedrich – Peaceful ruler

35. Gerda – Protected
36. Gerhard – Brave spear
37. Giselle – Pledge
38. Gustav – Staff of the Goths
39. Hannelore – Grace, light
40. Heinrich – Home ruler
41. Helga – Holy, blessed
42. Hermann – Army man
43. Hilda – Battle woman
44. Hugo – Mind, intellect
45. Ingrid – Beautiful
46. Isolde – Ice battle
47. Jakob – Supplanter
48. Johann – God is gracious
49. Jürgen – Earth-worker
50. Karl – Free man
51. Katarina – Pure
52. Klaus – Victory of the people
53. Konrad – Bold counsel
54. Leopold – Bold people
55. Liesel – God is my oath
56. Lina – Tender
57. Lorenz – Crowned with laurels
58. Ludwig – Famous warrior
59. Maja – Mother
60. Manfred – Man of peace
61. Margarete – Pearl
62. Maria – Bitter
63. Mathilda – Mighty in battle
64. Max – Greatest
65. Moritz – Dark-skinned
66. Nikolaus – Victory of the people
67. Otto – Wealth, fortune
68. Paul – Humble
69. Petra – Rock
70. Rainer – Wise army

71. Reinhard – Brave counsel
72. Rolf – Famous wolf
73. Rosa – Rose
74. Rudolf – Famous wolf
75. Sabine – Woman of the Sabine people
76. Siegfried – Victory peace
77. Sigrid – Beautiful victory
78. Sofia – Wisdom
79. Stefan – Crown
80. Theodor – Gift of God
81. Thomas – Twin
82. Udo – Wealthy
83. Ulrich – Power of the home
84. Ursula – Little bear
85. Valentin – Healthy, strong
86. Vera – Faith
87. Viktor – Conqueror
88. Walther – Ruler of the army
89. Wilhelm – Will, desire, helmet, protection
90. Wolfgang – Traveling wolf
91. Xavier – New house
92. Yvonne – Yew, archer
93. Zara – Princess
94. Zelda – Gray fighting maid
95. Annette – Grace
96. Bertram – Bright, raven
97. Christa – Follower of Christ
98. Dieter – Ruler of the people
99. Erika – Eternal ruler
100. Frauke – Little lady

French baby names and their meanings

1. Adrien - Dark One
2. Albert - Noble and Bright
3. Alexandre - Defender of Mankind
4. Alphonse - Ready for Battle
5. Andre - Manly
6. Antoine - Priceless One
7. Armand - Soldier
8. Augustin - Great
9. Baptiste - Baptist
10. Bastien - Revered
11. Benoit - Blessed
12. Bernard - Brave as a Bear
13. Blaise - Lisp, Stutter
14. Bruno - Brown
15. Camille - Young Ceremonial Attendant
16. Cedric - Bounty
17. Charles - Free Man
18. Claude - Lame
19. Clement - Merciful, Gentle
20. Damien - To Tame
21. Daniel - God is My Judge
22. Denis - Follower of Dionysius
23. Edouard - Wealthy Guardian
24. Emile - Rival
25. Etienne - Crown
26. Fabien - Bean Grower
27. Felix - Happy, Fortunate
28. Fernand - Adventurous, Courageous
29. Francois - Free Man
30. Gabriel - God is My Strength
31. Gaston - Guest, Stranger
32. Georges - Farmer
33. Gerard - Spear Brave
34. Gilbert - Bright Pledge

35. Gilles - Shield of Goatskin
36. Guillaume - Resolute Protector
37. Gustave - Staff of the Goths
38. Henri - Home Ruler
39. Herve - Army Warrior
40. Hubert - Bright Heart
41. Hugo - Mind, Intellect
42. Jacques - Supplanter
43. Jean - God is Gracious
44. Jerome - Sacred Name
45. Joachim - Established by God
46. Jules - Youthful, Downy
47. Laurent - Crowned with Laurels
48. Leon - Lion
49. Louis - Famous Warrior
50. Luc - Light
51. Marcel - Little Warrior
52. Mathieu - Gift of God
53. Maurice - Dark-Skinned, Moorish
54. Michel - Who is Like God?
55. Noel - Christmas
56. Olivier - Olive Tree
57. Pascal - Born on Easter
58. Patrice - Nobleman
59. Paul - Small
60. Philippe - Lover of Horses
61. Pierre - Rock
62. Quentin - Fifth
63. Raoul - Wolf Counsel
64. Raymond - Wise Protector
65. Rene - Reborn
66. Richard - Brave Ruler
67. Robert - Bright Fame
68. Romain - Roman
69. Serge - Servant
70. Simon - He has Heard

71. Stephane - Crown
72. Thierry - Ruler of the People
73. Thomas - Twin
74. Tristan - Tumult, Outcry
75. Valentin - Strong, Healthy
76. Victor - Conqueror
77. Vincent - Conquering
78. Xavier - New House
79. Yves - Yew Wood
80. Zoe - Life
81. Adele - Noble, Kind
82. Agathe - Good
83. Aimee - Beloved
84. Amelie - Hardworking
85. Anais - Grace
86. Beatrice - She who brings happiness
87. Camille - Young ceremonial attendant
88. Celeste - Heavenly
89. Charlotte - Free woman
90. Chloe - Blooming
91. Claire - Clear, Bright
92. Colette - People of Victory
93. Danielle - God is My Judge
94. Eloise - Healthy, Wide
95. Emmanuelle - God is with Us
96. Fleur - Flower
97. Gabrielle - God is My Strength
98. Helene - Shining Light
99. Isabelle - God is My Oath
100. Josephine - God Will Add

Italian baby names and their meanings

1. Alessandro - Defender of mankind
2. Bianca - White or pure
3. Carlo - Free man
4. Dario - Possessor of good
5. Elena - Shining light
6. Federico - Peaceful ruler
7. Gianna - The Lord is gracious
8. Hugo - Mind, intellect
9. Isabella - Devoted to God
10. Jacopo - Supplanter
11. Katerina - Pure
12. Lorenzo - From Laurentum, Italy
13. Maria - Sea of sorrow
14. Nicola - Victory of the people
15. Orlando - Famous land
16. Piero - Rock
17. Quirino - Warlike
18. Raffaello - God has healed
19. Serena - Calm, tranquil
20. Tommaso - Twin
21. Umberto - Bright bear
22. Valentina - Strength, health
23. Zaira - Rose
24. Adriano - From Hadria
25. Beatrice - She who brings happiness
26. Claudia - Lame
27. Dante - Lasting, enduring
28. Emilia - Rival
29. Fabio - Bean grower
30. Giulia - Youthful
31. Ida - Industrious one
32. Leonardo - Brave lion
33. Marco - Warlike
34. Nicoletta - Victory of the people

35. Ottavia - Eighth
36. Paolo - Small or humble
37. Riccardo - Powerful ruler
38. Sofia - Wisdom
39. Tiziano - Giant
40. Ugo - Mind, intellect
41. Vittoria - Victory
42. Zeno - Gift of Zeus
43. Alessia - Defender
44. Bernardo - Brave as a bear
45. Chiara - Bright, clear
46. Domenico - Belonging to the Lord
47. Elisa - God is my oath
48. Francesco - Free man
49. Gabriella - God is my strength
50. Ilario - Cheerful
51. Jacinta - Hyacinth
52. Luca - Light
53. Matteo - Gift of God
54. Noemi - Pleasantness
55. Orazio - Timekeeper
56. Pietro - Rock
57. Rosalia - Rose
58. Stefano - Crown
59. Teodoro - Gift of God
60. Umbria - Shadow
61. Veronica - True image
62. Angelo - Messenger of God
63. Bruna - Brown-haired
64. Cosimo - Order, beauty
65. Donatella - Beautiful gift
66. Ettore - Loyal
67. Fabrizio - Craftsman
68. Giorgio - Farmer
69. Isidoro - Gift of Isis
70. Ludovico - Famous warrior

71. Marcella - Warlike
72. Natalia - Born on Christmas Day
73. Olga - Holy
74. Primo - First
75. Renata - Reborn
76. Silvia - From the forest
77. Tullio - Peaceful
78. Vincenzo - Conquering
79. Zita - Little girl
80. Amadeo - Love of God
81. Benedetta - Blessed
82. Cesare - Hairy
83. Delfina - Dolphin
84. Ernesto - Serious, resolute
85. Filippo - Friend of horses
86. Giuliano - Youthful
87. Ippolito - Horse freer
88. Livia - Envious
89. Massimo - Greatest
90. Novella - New
91. Olimpia - From Olympus
92. Pia - Pious
93. Rosario - Rosary
94. Salvatore - Savior
95. Teresa - Harvester
96. Uberto - Bright mind
97. Valeria - To be strong
98. Alessa - Defender
99. Berto - Bright, famous
100. Chiara - Clear, bright

Spanish baby names and their meanings

1. Alejandro – Defender
2. Alondra – Lark
3. Adelina – Noble
4. Adrián – From Hadria
5. Amalia – Hardworking
6. Antonio – Priceless
7. Araceli – Altar of the sky
8. Beatriz – Bringer of joy
9. Benito – Blessed
10. Blanca – White
11. Camila – Perfect
12. Carlos – Free man
13. Carmen – Song
14. Consuelo – Comfort
15. Cristóbal – Christ-bearer
16. Dolores – Sorrows
17. Diego – Supplanter
18. Emilio – Rival
19. Esperanza – Hope
20. Esteban – Crown
21. Fernanda – Adventurous
22. Francisco – Free man
23. Gabriela – God is my strength
24. Gerardo – Spear rule
25. Hector – Holding fast
26. Ignacio – Fiery
27. Isabela – Devoted to God
28. Javier – New house
29. Jose – God will increase
30. Juan – God is gracious
31. Julio – Youthful
32. Laura – Laurel
33. Lucia – Light
34. Luis – Famous warrior

35. Manuel – God is with us
36. Maria – Bitter
37. Marta – Lady
38. Miguel – Who is like God?
39. Natalia – Born on Christmas day
40. Olivia – Olive tree
41. Pablo – Small
42. Patricia – Noble
43. Rafael – God has healed
44. Ramon – Wise protector
45. Ricardo – Powerful ruler
46. Roberto – Bright fame
47. Rosa – Rose
48. Santiago – Saint James
49. Sofia – Wisdom
50. Teresa – Harvester
51. Valeria – Strength
52. Victor – Conqueror
53. Yolanda – Violet flower
54. Zacarias – God has remembered
55. Abel – Breath
56. Adan – Earth
57. Agustin – Majestic
58. Alba – Dawn
59. Andres – Manly
60. Angel – Messenger of God
61. Aurora – Dawn
62. Belen – Bethlehem
63. Bruno – Brown
64. Cecilia – Blind
65. Clara – Clear, bright
66. Daniel – God is my judge
67. David – Beloved
68. Elena – Shining light
69. Eva – Life
70. Felipe – Friend of horses

71. Gloria – Glory
72. Guillermo – Will helmet
73. Hugo – Mind, intellect
74. Ines – Chaste
75. Joaquin – God will judge
76. Karina – Pure
77. Leon – Lion
78. Mariana – Grace
79. Noemi – My delight
80. Oscar – Divine spear
81. Paloma – Dove
82. Raquel – Ewe
83. Samuel – God has heard
84. Susana – Lily
85. Tomas – Twin
86. Ursula – Little bear
87. Veronica – True image
88. Ximena – Hearkening
89. Yasmin – Jasmine flower
90. Zara – Princess
91. Abelardo – Resolute
92. Adela – Noble
93. Bonita – Pretty
94. Cesar – Long haired
95. Dulce – Sweet
96. Enrique – Home ruler
97. Fabiana – Bean grower
98. Gracia – Grace
99. Isidro – Gifted with many ideas
100. Jacinta – Hyacinth

Chinese baby names and their meanings

1. Li – Beautiful
2. Wang – King
3. Zhang – Archer
4. Liu – Kill, Destroy
5. Chen – Great
6. Yang – Poplar Tree
7. Huang – Yellow
8. Zhao – Enlightened
9. Wu – Martial
10. Zhou – State
11. Xu – Slow
12. Sun – Obedient
13. Ma – Horse
14. Zhu – Vermilion; Bright
15. Hu – Tiger
16. Guo – Country
17. Lin – Forest
18. He – Crane
19. Gao – High, Tall
20. Luo – Camel
21. Song – Pine Tree
22. Zheng – Upright, Honest
23. Tian – Sky
24. Dong – East
25. Peng – Roc (a mythical bird)
26. Cai – Wealth
27. Cui – Green
28. Zeng – Increase
29. Han – Korean
30. Shen – Deep
31. Ou – Lotus
32. Fang – Fragrant
33. Yuan – Original
34. Zou – Walk

35. Bai – White
36. Bao – Treasure
37. Ding – Nail
38. Tian – Field
39. Jiang – River
40. Qiu – Autumn
41. Wei – Guard
42. You – Excellent
43. Xie – Thank You
44. Liao – Chat
45. Jin – Gold
46. Yao – Distant
47. Yue – Moon
48. Tong – Bronze
49. Shao – Young
50. Miao – Wonderful
51. Lei – Thunder
52. Zhuo – Bright
53. Bao – Jewel
54. Min – Quick
55. Qin – Zither
56. Fang – Square
57. Xiong – Bear
58. Jian – Healthy
59. Tao – Peach
60. Qiang – Strong
61. Du – Capital
62. Pan – Hope
63. Dai – Black
64. Xia – Summer
65. Shang – Appreciate
66. Ping – Peaceful
67. Yu – Jade
68. Rong – Glory
69. Yuan – Round
70. Mao – Fur

71. Ning – Tranquil
72. Qian – Money
73. Xiu – Elegant
74. Chai – Firewood
75. Jing – Quiet
76. Cheng – Accomplish
77. Teng – Soaring
78. Xun – Fast
79. Yue – Music
80. Zhen – Precious
81. Hao – Good
82. Xing – Star
83. Lian – Lotus
84. Shen – Spirit
85. Lu – Deer
86. Lang – Wolf
87. Yong – Brave
88. Hui – Bright
89. Qi – Enlighten
90. Jia – Good
91. Su – Plain
92. Zhi – Wisdom
93. Huan – Joy
94. Shui – Water
95. Bing – Ice
96. Feng – Wind
97. Huo – Fire
98. Shan – Mountain
99. Kuo – Expand
100. An – Peace

Japanese baby names and their meanings

1. Aiko – Beloved child
2. Akemi – Bright and beautiful
3. Amaya – Night rain
4. Asuka – Tomorrow's fragrance
5. Chiyo – Thousand generations
6. Emiko – Blessed child
7. Fumiko – Child of abundant beauty
8. Haruka – Far-off
9. Hikari – Light
10. Izumi – Fountain, spring
11. Junko – Pure child
12. Kaori – Fragrance
13. Kimiko – Noble child
14. Maiko – Dancing child
15. Miyuki – Beautiful happiness
16. Naoko – Honest child
17. Noriko – Lawful child
18. Rina – Jasmine
19. Sachiko – Happy child
20. Tomoko – Wise child
21. Yumi – Beauty
22. Yuriko – Lily child
23. Akio – Bright man
24. Daiki – Great glory
25. Eiji – Eternity
26. Fumio – Scholarly hero
27. Haruki – Shining sun
28. Isamu – Courage
29. Junichi – Obedient one
30. Kaito – Ocean flying
31. Makoto – Sincerity
32. Naoki – Honest tree
33. Osamu – Discipline, study
34. Ryo – Cool, refreshing

35. Satoshi – Wise, fast learner
36. Takumi – Artisan
37. Yori – Trust
38. Yuji – Courageous second son
39. Hiroshi – Generous
40. Ichiro – First son
41. Kazuki – Harmonious hope
42. Kenji – Strong and vigorous
43. Masaru – Victory
44. Nobu – Faith
45. Ren – Lotus
46. Shin – Genuine, real
47. Toshi – Wise
48. Yoshi – Good luck
49. Yuki – Snow
50. Hideki – Excellent timber
51. Kiyoshi – Pure
52. Yoshio – Righteous man
53. Yasu – Peace
54. Kei – Blessing
55. Sora – Sky
56. Riku – Land
57. Hinata – Sunny place
58. Itsuki – Tree
59. Asahi – Morning sun
60. Youta – Great sunlight
61. Madoka – Circle, round
62. Sakura – Cherry blossom
63. Hana – Flower
64. Ayame – Iris
65. Yui – Tie, bind
66. Aoi – Hollyhock, blue
67. Mio – Beautiful cherry blossom
68. Riko – Jasmine child
69. Sumire – Violet
70. Sayuri – Little lily

71. Shizuka – Quiet
72. Mariko – True village child
73. Nanami – Seven seas
74. Misaki – Beautiful blossom
75. Yukari – Beautiful pear tree
76. Saki – Blossom of hope
77. Nozomi – Hope
78. Minori – Beautiful harbor
79. Rei – Beautiful
80. Kana – Powerful
81. Natsuki – Summer hope
82. Miku – Beautiful sky
83. Ayaka – Colorful flower
84. Chieko – Child of intelligence
85. Etsuko – Joyful child
86. Hideko – Child of excellence
87. Iku – Nourishing
88. Kazuko – Child of harmony
89. Kumiko – Long-time beautiful child
90. Midori – Green
91. Natsuko – Summer child
92. Reiko – Grateful child
93. Setsuko – Temperate child
94. Tamiko – Child of many beauties
95. Yuko – Gentle child
96. Yoko – Positive child
97. Akane – Brilliant red
98. Maki – True hope
99. Yuri – Lily
100. Yoko – Child of sunlight

Indian baby names and their meanings

1. Aarav - Peaceful
2. Vihaan - Dawn
3. Arjun - Bright, Shining
4. Vivaan - Full of life
5. Aditya - Sun
6. Aryan - Noble
7. Dhruv - Pole star
8. Atharv - First Veda
9. Advait - Unique
10. Ishaan - Sun
11. Aarush - First ray of the sun
12. Aadi - Beginning
13. Rudra - Lord Shiva
14. Aahan - Dawn
15. Kavish - Poet
16. Hrithik - From the heart
17. Rehan - Scented
18. Ayaan - Good luck
19. Aaradhya - Worshipped
20. Aanya - Limitless
21. Anaya - Caring
22. Aadhya - First power
23. Kiara - Bright
24. Diya - Light
25. Kavya - Poetry
26. Aarna - Goddess Lakshmi
27. Aahana - First rays of the sun
28. Saanvi - Goddess Lakshmi
29. Myra - Sweet, Admirable
30. Shanaya - First ray of the sun
31. Anika - Grace
32. Sara - Pure, Happy
33. Alisha - Protected by God
34. Riya - Singer

35. Navya - New, Young
36. Aarohi - A music tune
37. Prisha - God's gift
38. Ananya - Unique
39. Pari - Fairy
40. Kaira - Peaceful
41. Avni - Earth
42. Ayesha - Lively
43. Ahana - Inner light
44. Anushka - Grace
45. Ishita - Superior
46. Aditi - Freedom, Boundless
47. Aaravi - Peace
48. Aashi - Smile, Joy
49. Aarna - Goddess Lakshmi
50. Aarini - Adventurous
51. Aahna - Exist
52. Aarika - Adored
53. Aashna - Beloved
54. Amaaya - Night rain
55. Aanya - Inexhaustible
56. Aarshi - Heavenly
57. Aarini - Brave
58. Aarabi - Singing
59. Aarunya - First rays of the sun
60. Aaratrika - Dusk lamp beneath 'Tulsi' plant
61. Aarika - Admired for looks
62. Aarohi - Evolving
63. Aashita - One who is hopeful
64. Aarushi - First rays of the sun
65. Aishani - Goddess Durga
66. Aaradhya - Worship
67. Aashi - Blessings
68. Aarini - Adventurous
69. Aakanksha - Desire, Wish
70. Aaratrika - The Dusk Lamp beneath 'Tulsi' plant

71. Aakriti - Shape
72. Aanya - Grace
73. Aarohi - A music tune
74. Aashna - Hope
75. Aarna - Lakshmi
76. Aarushi - First rays of the sun
77. Aastha - Faith
78. Aahna - Exist
79. Aabha - Glow, Luster
80. Aadrika - Mountain
81. Aaradhya - Worship
82. Aahana - Inner light
83. Aanya - Inexhaustible
84. Aarika - Adored
85. Aarshi - Heavenly
86. Aarini - Adventurous
87. Aarabi - Singing
88. Aarunya - First rays of the sun
89. Aaratrika - Dusk lamp beneath 'Tulsi' plant
90. Aarika - Admired for looks
91. Aarohi - Evolving
92. Aashita - One who is hopeful
93. Aarushi - First rays of the sun
94. Aishani - Goddess Durga
95. Aaradhya - Worship
96. Aashi - Blessings
97. Aarini - Adventurous
98. Aakanksha - Desire, Wish
99. Aaratrika - The Dusk Lamp beneath 'Tulsi' plant
100. Aakriti - Shape

Mexican baby names and their meanings

1. Adela – Noble
2. Adriana – Dark
3. Agustina – Majestic
4. Alberto – Noble and Bright
5. Alejandro – Defender of mankind
6. Alicia – Noble
7. Alonzo – Ready for battle
8. Alvaro – Guardian
9. Amada – Beloved
10. Amado – Loved one
11. Ana – Grace
12. Andres – Manly
13. Angel – Messenger of God
14. Antonia – Priceless
15. Antonio – Priceless
16. Araceli – Altar of heaven
17. Arturo – Bear
18. Beatriz – Bringer of joy
19. Benito – Blessed
20. Blanca – White
21. Camila – Perfect
22. Carlos – Free man
23. Carmen – Song
24. Cesar – Long-haired
25. Clara – Bright, clear
26. Concepcion – Conception
27. Consuelo – Consolation
28. Cristian – Follower of Christ
29. Cristina – Follower of Christ
30. Daniel – God is my judge
31. Diego – Supplanter
32. Dolores – Sorrows
33. Eduardo – Wealthy guardian
34. Elena – Shining light

35. Emilio – Rival
36. Enrique – Home ruler
37. Ernesto – Serious
38. Esmeralda – Emerald
39. Esteban – Crown
40. Eva – Life
41. Felipe – Lover of horses
42. Fernando – Adventurous
43. Francisco – Free man
44. Gabriel – God is my strength
45. Gloria – Glory
46. Graciela – Grace
47. Guillermo – Resolute protector
48. Hector – Holding fast
49. Hugo – Mind, intellect
50. Ignacio – Fiery
51. Inez – Pure
52. Isabel – God's promise
53. Javier – Bright
54. Jesus – God is salvation
55. Joaquin – God will establish
56. Jorge – Farmer
57. Jose – God will increase
58. Juan – God is gracious
59. Juana – God is gracious
60. Julio – Youthful
61. Laura – Laurel
62. Leon – Lion
63. Leonardo – Brave lion
64. Lourdes – From Lourdes, France
65. Lucia – Light
66. Luis – Famous warrior
67. Manuel – God is with us
68. Marcela – Young warrior
69. Marco – Warlike
70. Maria – Sea of bitterness

71. Mario – Warlike
72. Marta – Lady
73. Martin – Warlike
74. Miguel – Who is like God?
75. Natalia – Born on Christmas Day
76. Nicolas – Victory of the people
77. Olivia – Olive tree
78. Oscar – God's spear
79. Pablo – Small
80. Patricia – Noble
81. Pedro – Rock
82. Pilar – Pillar
83. Rafael – God has healed
84. Ramon – Wise protector
85. Raquel – Ewe
86. Ricardo – Strong ruler
87. Roberto – Bright fame
88. Rosa – Rose
89. Salvador – Savior
90. Santiago – Supplanter
91. Sara – Princess
92. Sergio – Servant
93. Sofia – Wisdom
94. Teresa – Harvester
95. Tomas – Twin
96. Veronica – True image
97. Victor – Conqueror
98. Victoria – Victory
99. Vincente – Conquering
100. Yolanda – Violet flower

Brazilian baby names and their meanings

1. Adriana – Dark
2. Alessandra – Defender of mankind
3. Andre – Manly, brave
4. Antonio – Priceless one
5. Beatriz – She who brings joy
6. Bernardo – Brave as a bear
7. Bruna – Brown-haired
8. Camila – Young ceremonial attendant
9. Carlos – Free man
10. Cecilia – Blind
11. Clara – Clear, bright
12. Daniel – God is my judge
13. Eduardo – Wealthy guardian
14. Elisa – God is my oath
15. Fabio – Bean grower
16. Gabriel – God is my strength
17. Helena – Light
18. Isabela – Devoted to God
19. Joao – God is gracious
20. Julia – Youthful
21. Leonardo – Brave lion
22. Lucas – Light
23. Maria – Bitter
24. Marina – Of the sea
25. Natalia – Born on Christmas
26. Olivia – Olive tree
27. Paulo – Small
28. Rafael – God has healed
29. Sofia – Wisdom
30. Tiago – Supplanter
31. Vanessa – Butterfly
32. Victor – Conqueror
33. Yasmin – Jasmine flower
34. Zara – Princess

35. Ana – Gracious
36. Bruno – Brown
37. Carolina – Free woman
38. Davi – Beloved
39. Estela – Star
40. Felipe – Friend of horses
41. Guilherme – Will helmet
42. Isabel – Pledged to God
43. Joana – God is gracious
44. Kaio – Rejoice
45. Larissa – Cheerful
46. Mateus – Gift of God
47. Nicole – Victory of the people
48. Otavio – Eighth
49. Patricia – Noble
50. Ricardo – Powerful ruler
51. Samuel – God has heard
52. Teresa – Harvester
53. Uriel – God is my light
54. Viviane – Alive
55. Wilson – Son of Will
56. Ximena – Listening
57. Yara – Water lady
58. Zacarias – God remembers
59. Abel – Breath
60. Bianca – White
61. Cristiano – Follower of Christ
62. Denise – Devotee of Dionysus
63. Elias – The Lord is my God
64. Fernanda – Adventurous, brave journey
65. Gustavo – Staff of the Goths
66. Iris – Rainbow
67. Jessica – God beholds
68. Kevin – Gentle birth
69. Livia – Envious
70. Marcos – Warlike

71. Noemi – Pleasantness
72. Oscar – Divine spear
73. Priscila – Ancient
74. Rebeca – To tie
75. Silvia – Woodland
76. Tadeu – Heart
77. Ursula – Little bear
78. Valentina – Strong, healthy
79. Wilma – Will, desire
80. Xavier – New house
81. Yves – Yew
82. Zacarias – God has remembered
83. Amanda – Worthy of love
84. Bruno – Brown
85. Cecilia – Blind
86. Diego – Supplanter
87. Esther – Star
88. Fabiana – Bean grower
89. Gabriel – God is my strength
90. Heitor – Holding fast
91. Ines – Pure
92. Juliana – Youthful
93. Karina – Pure
94. Lucas – Light
95. Mariana – Bitter grace
96. Natan – Given
97. Olivia – Olive tree
98. Pedro – Rock
99. Raquel – Ewe
100. Sergio – Servant

Russian baby names and their meanings

1. Anastasia - Resurrection
2. Alexei - Defender
3. Andrei - Manly
4. Anna - Grace
5. Anton - Priceless
6. Boris - Fighter
7. Daria - Wealthy
8. Dmitri - Earth-lover
9. Ekaterina - Pure
10. Elena - Shining light
11. Feodor - Gift of God
12. Galina - Calm
13. Grigori - Watchful
14. Igor - Warrior of peace
15. Irina - Peace
16. Ivan - God is gracious
17. Kira - Leader
18. Konstantin - Constant
19. Larisa - Cheerful
20. Leonid - Lion-like
21. Maria - Wished-for child
22. Maxim - Greatest
23. Natalia - Born on Christmas Day
24. Nikita - Unconquerable
25. Olga - Holy
26. Pavel - Small
27. Sergei - Servant
28. Sofia - Wisdom
29. Tatiana - Fairy queen
30. Valentin - Strong, healthy
31. Valeria - Strength
32. Vladimir - Ruler of the world
33. Yelena - Bright, shining light
34. Yuri - Farmer

35. Zoya - Life
36. Aleksandr - Defender of mankind
37. Alina - Bright, beautiful
38. Anastasiya - Resurrection
39. Angelina - Messenger of God
40. Artyom - Safe and sound
41. Dasha - Gift of God
42. Evgeni - Noble
43. Fyodor - Gift of God
44. Gleb - Heir
45. Inna - Strong water
46. Katya - Pure
47. Lilia - Lily
48. Maksim - Greatest
49. Nadya - Hope
50. Oksana - Praise be to God
51. Polina - Small
52. Ruslan - Lion man
53. Svetlana - Light
54. Timur - Iron
55. Vasilisa - Queen
56. Viktor - Conqueror
57. Yana - God is gracious
58. Zhenya - Noble
59. Zhanna - God is gracious
60. Kirill - Lord
61. Lyudmila - Love of the people
62. Mila - Gracious
63. Nadia - Hope
64. Oleg - Holy
65. Pyotr - Rock
66. Raisa - Easy-going
67. Stanislav - Glory
68. Tatyana - Fairy queen
69. Vanya - God is gracious
70. Yaroslav - Fierce and glorious

71. Zhanna - God is merciful
72. Danila - God is my judge
73. Elizaveta - God's promise
74. Fedor - Divine gift
75. Gavriil - God is my strength
76. Ilya - The Lord is my God
77. Klara - Bright, clear
78. Lada - Goddess of beauty and fertility
79. Miroslav - Peace and glory
80. Nastya - Resurrection
81. Olesya - Defender
82. Radomir - Happy peace
83. Serafima - Burning one
84. Taisiya - Bandage
85. Vasilisa - Queen
86. Yulia - Youthful
87. Zlata - Golden
88. Aleksey - Defender
89. Bogdan - Gift from God
90. Dima - Earth mother
91. Evdokia - Good seeming
92. Grisha - Watchful
93. Irina - Peace
94. Kolya - People's victory
95. Lyubov - Love
96. Misha - Who is like God?
97. Natasha - Born on Christmas Day
98. Olya - Holy
99. Rostislav - Usurp glory
100. Sveta - Light

Dutch baby names and their meanings

1. Abel – Breath
2. Adriaan – From Hadria
3. Aart – Like an eagle
4. Bastiaan – Venerable
5. Bram – Father of many
6. Cas – Imperial
7. Daan – God is my judge
8. Dirk – Ruler of the people
9. Evert – Strong as a boar
10. Frits – Peaceful ruler
11. Gijs – Bright pledge
12. Hans – God is gracious
13. Ivo – Yew
14. Joost – Just
15. Kees – Horn
16. Leendert – Lion strength
17. Maarten – From Mars
18. Noud – Wealthy, powerful
19. Otto – Wealth
20. Piet – Rock
21. Quinten – Fifth
22. Roel – Famous land
23. Stijn – Constant
24. Teun – Priceless, inestimable
25. Udo – Prosperous, rich
26. Vincent – Conquering
27. Wim – With helmet
28. Xander – Defender of the people
29. Yorick – Farmer
30. Zeger – Victory bearer
31. Aafke – Noble, kind
32. Babette – Stranger, traveller
33. Carina – Dear, beloved
34. Doutzen – Dove

35. Elsje – Noble, kind
36. Femke – Peaceful ruler
37. Grietje – Pearl
38. Hanne – God's gracious gift
39. Inge – Ing is beautiful
40. Jolijn – Violet
41. Katrien – Pure
42. Liesbeth – God's promise
43. Machteld – Powerful in battle
44. Nienke – Clean, pure
45. Odette – Wealth
46. Petra – Rock
47. Quinty – Fifth
48. Roos – Rose
49. Sophie – Wisdom
50. Tessa – Harvester
51. Ursula – Little bear
52. Vera – Faith
53. Willemijn – Will, desire, helmet, protection
54. Xandra – Defender of the people
55. Yvette – Yew
56. Zara – Princess
57. Arie – Lion of God
58. Berend – Brave as a bear
59. Coen – Bold, brave
60. Diederik – Ruler of the people
61. Eelco – Noble, famous
62. Frans – Free man
63. Gerard – Brave spear
64. Hendrik – Home ruler
65. IJsbrand – Ice sword
66. Jaap – Supplanter
67. Klaas – Victory of the people
68. Laurens – From Laurentum
69. Michel – Who is like God?
70. Niels – Champion

71. Olivier – Olive tree
72. Paul – Small, humble
73. Rik – Powerful ruler
74. Sander – Defender of the people
75. Thijs – Gift of God
76. Victor – Conqueror
77. Wouter – Army ruler
78. Xavi – New house
79. Yannick – God is gracious
80. Zoe – Life
81. Anouk – Grace, mercy
82. Beatrix – She who brings happiness
83. Celine – Heavenly
84. Desiree – Desired
85. Eva – Life
86. Fleur – Flower
87. Hilda – Battle woman
88. Iris – Rainbow
89. Julia – Youthful, downy
90. Karlijn – Free man
91. Lotte – Free man
92. Marit – Pearl
93. Noor – Light
94. Pien – God will add
95. Rianne – Queen
96. Sanne – Lily
97. Tineke – Follower of Christ
98. Veerle – Travel, protection
99. Willeke – Will, desire, helmet, protection
100. Yara – Small butterfly

Swedish baby names and their meanings

1. Agnes – Pure or holy
2. Albin – White or bright
3. Alice – Noble
4. Alva – Elf
5. Anders – Manly or brave
6. Anna – Grace or favor
7. Anton – Priceless
8. Arvid – Eagle tree
9. Astrid – Beautiful goddess
10. Axel – Father of peace
11. Beatrice – She who brings happiness
12. Birgitta – Strong or exalted one
13. Bjorn – Bear
14. Carl – Free man
15. Cecilia – Blind
16. Clara – Bright or clear
17. Dag – Day
18. Ebba – Strong
19. Edvin – Rich friend
20. Elin – Shining light
21. Elsa – God's promise
22. Emil – Rival
23. Emma – Universal
24. Erik – Eternal ruler
25. Ester – Star
26. Felix – Happy or fortunate
27. Filip – Lover of horses
28. Fredrik – Peaceful ruler
29. Frida – Peace
30. Gabriel – God is my strength
31. Gustav – Staff of the gods
32. Hanna – Grace
33. Harald – Army ruler
34. Hedvig – Battle maiden

35. Helena – Light
36. Hugo – Mind or intellect
37. Ida – Work
38. Ingrid – Beautiful
39. Isak – He will laugh
40. Jakob – Supplanter
41. Johan – God is gracious
42. Julia – Youthful
43. Karl – Free man
44. Klara – Clear or bright
45. Kristian – Follower of Christ
46. Lennart – Lion strength
47. Lina – Tender
48. Linnea – Lime tree
49. Ludvig – Famous warrior
50. Lukas – From Lucania
51. Maja – Mother
52. Malin – High tower
53. Marcus – Warlike
54. Maria – Wished-for child
55. Martin – Warlike
56. Matilda – Battle-mighty
57. Mikael – Who is like God?
58. Nils – Champion
59. Oskar – Friend of deer
60. Otto – Wealth or fortune
61. Paula – Small
62. Pernilla – Rock
63. Peter – Rock
64. Ragnar – Army advice
65. Rasmus – Beloved
66. Rebecca – To tie or bind
67. Robert – Bright fame
68. Roger – Famous spear
69. Rosa – Rose
70. Samuel – God has heard

71. Sara – Princess
72. Sebastian – Venerable
73. Sigrid – Beautiful victory
74. Sofia – Wisdom
75. Stefan – Crown
76. Stina – Christian
77. Sven – Boy, lad
78. Tilda – Battle-mighty
79. Tomas – Twin
80. Ulf – Wolf
81. Ulrika – Ruler of all
82. Valdemar – Famous ruler
83. Vera – Faith
84. Viktor – Conqueror
85. Vilma – Resolute protector
86. Vincent – Conquering
87. Wilhelm – Will-helmet
88. Ylva – She-wolf
89. Yngve – The god Ing
90. Ake – Ancestor
91. Edith – Prosperous in war
92. Gunilla – Battle maiden
93. Ingmar – Famous son
94. Leif – Heir or descendant
95. Magdalena – Woman from Magdala
96. Nanna – Brave
97. Orjan – Farmer
98. Rolf – Famous wolf
99. Tove – Beautiful Thor
100. Viveka – Little woman

Norwegian baby names and their meanings

1. Aksel – Father of Peace
2. Anja – Grace
3. Arne – Eagle
4. Astrid – Divinely Beautiful
5. Birgit – The Exalted One
6. Bjorn – Bear
7. Dag – Day
8. Einar – One Warrior
9. Elsa – God's Promise
10. Emil – Rival
11. Frida – Peace
12. Greta – Pearl
13. Hakon – High Son
14. Ida – Industrious One
15. Ingrid – Beautiful
16. Jens – God is Gracious
17. Kari – Pure
18. Lars – Crowned with Laurel
19. Magnus – Great
20. Nils – Champion
21. Ola – Ancestor's Descendant
22. Petra – Rock
23. Reidar – Home Warrior
24. Sigrid – Beautiful Victory
25. Tore – Thunder God
26. Unn – Love
27. Vebjorn – Sacred Bear
28. Ylva – She-Wolf
29. Zara – Princess
30. Alf – Elf Counsel
31. Bente – Blessed
32. Casper – Treasurer
33. Dagny – New Day
34. Edvard – Wealthy Guardian

35. Freja – Lady, Noblewoman
36. Gunner – Bold Warrior
37. Hilde – Battle
38. Isak – Laughter
39. Johanne – God is Gracious
40. Kjell – Helmet
41. Leif – Heir, Descendant
42. Maren – Sea
43. Nora – Honor
44. Orjan – Farmer
45. Peder – Rock
46. Ragna – Advice, Counsel
47. Siv – Bride
48. Tordis – Thor's Goddess
49. Ulrik – Prosperity and Power
50. Vidar – Warrior
51. Agnete – Pure, Holy
52. Bjarte – Bright
53. Cecilie – Blind
54. Dagfinn – Day, Finn
55. Eirik – Eternal Ruler
56. Fridtjof – Thief of Peace
57. Gro – To Grow
58. Hakon – High Son
59. Inge – Ancestor
60. Jan – God is Gracious
61. Katarina – Pure
62. Lars – Crowned with Laurel
63. Marit – Pearl
64. Njord – Strong
65. Odd – Tip of the Blade
66. Per – Rock
67. Rolf – Famous Wolf
68. Stian – Wanderer
69. Tove – Beautiful Thor
70. Ulf – Wolf

71. Vilhelm – Determined Protector
72. Alette – Noble
73. Bjorg – Help, Salvation
74. Carina – Dear, Beloved
75. Dagmar – Day's Glory
76. Elin – Light
77. Frode – Wise
78. Gunnar – Warrior
79. Hilda – Battle
80. Ingeborg – Protection
81. Jorgen – Farmer
82. Knut – Knot
83. Lene – Torch
84. Marte – Lady
85. Nils – Victory of the People
86. Oskar – Friend of Deer
87. Pia – Pious
88. Roald – Famous Ruler
89. Sindre – Travelling
90. Tor – Thunder
91. Valdemar – Famous Ruler
92. Agnes – Pure
93. Bjorn – Bear
94. Charlotte – Free
95. Dagrun – Day's Secret Love
96. Erling – Descendant
97. Fredrik – Peaceful Ruler
98. Gudrun – God's Secret Love
99. Halvard – Defender of the Rock
100. Ingvild – Ing's Warrior

Danish baby names and their meanings

1. Aksel – Father of peace
2. Anders – Strong and manly
3. Anika – Grace
4. Asta – Love
5. Asger – Spear of God
6. Birgitte – The exalted one
7. Bodil – Commanding battle
8. Carsten – Christian
9. Dagmar – Maiden of the day
10. Einar – One warrior
11. Elsa – God's promise
12. Emil – Rival
13. Erik – Eternal ruler
14. Freja – Lady
15. Gerda – Enclosure
16. Grethe – Pearl
17. Hans – God is gracious
18. Henrik – Ruler of the home
19. Ingrid – Beautiful
20. Jakob – Supplanter
21. Jens – God is gracious
22. Jorgen – Farmer
23. Karsten – Anointed
24. Kirsten – Christian
25. Lars – Laurel
26. Lene – Torch
27. Magnus – Great
28. Mette – Pearl
29. Nils – Victory of the people
30. Olaf – Ancestor's descendant
31. Pernille – Rock
32. Rasmus – Beloved
33. Soren – Stern
34. Svend – Boy

35. Thyra – God's strength
36. Tobias – God is good
37. Ulf – Wolf
38. Viggo – War
39. Yvonne – Yew
40. Zita – Little girl
41. Abel – Breath
42. Bente – Blessed
43. Claus – Victory of the people
44. Dorte – Gift of God
45. Ebbe – Wild boar
46. Fiona – White
47. Gustav – Staff of the gods
48. Hanne – Grace
49. Ida – Hardworking
50. Jesper – Treasurer
51. Kaj – Rejoice
52. Leif – Heir
53. Mads – Gift from God
54. Nanna – Daring
55. Otto – Wealthy
56. Poul – Small
57. Rune – Secret
58. Stine – Christian
59. Tove – Beautiful Thor
60. Ulrik – Wealthy and powerful
61. Vibeke – Little woman
62. Yrsa – Wild bear
63. Aage – Ancestor
64. Britta – Strength
65. Casper – Treasurer
66. Ditte – Gift of God
67. Esben – Bear
68. Frida – Peace
69. Gunner – Warrior
70. Helle – Holy

71. Inge – Ing is beautiful
72. Jeppe – Supplanter
73. Kai – Rejoice
74. Lise – God's promise
75. Mogens – Power
76. Niels – Victory of the people
77. Oskar – Friend of deer
78. Pia – Pious
79. Rolf – Famous wolf
80. Signe – New victory
81. Thora – Thunder goddess
82. Ulla – Will, determination
83. Vilhelm – Will, desire and helmet, protection
84. Yngve – Son of Ing
85. Agnete – Holy, pure
86. Bjarne – Bear
87. Connie – Steadfastness
88. Dorthe – Gift of God
89. Egon – Edge of a sword
90. Frede – Peace
91. Gregers – Watchful, alert
92. Hilda – Battle woman
93. Ib – Yew
94. Jes – God will add
95. Keld – Spring, fountain
96. Lisbeth – God's promise
97. Maja – Mother
98. Nete – Pure, holy
99. Olga – Holy
100. Peder – Stone

Finnish baby names and their meanings

1. Aada – Noble
2. Aalto – Wave
3. Aamu – Morning
4. Aava – Open, Spacious
5. Aino – The Only One
6. Akseli – My Father is Peace
7. Alvar – Elf Warrior
8. Anja – Grace
9. Anneli – Grace and Light
10. Antti – Priceless One
11. Arja – Harvest
12. Arto – Bear, Stone
13. Asko – God's Gift
14. Eeli – My God is Yahweh
15. Eero – Forever Strong
16. Eetu – Wealthy Guardian
17. Eeva – Life
18. Eija – Merciful
19. Eino – Lone Warrior
20. Elina – Torch of Light
21. Ella – All, Completely
22. Elli – My God is an Oath
23. Elmo – Helmet, Protection
24. Elsa – Noble
25. Emil – Rival, Emulating
26. Erkki – Ever Ruler
27. Esa – God is Salvation
28. Essi – Star
29. Eveliina – Life
30. Haakon – High Son
31. Hanna – Grace
32. Harri – Home Ruler
33. Heikki – Home Ruler
34. Helena – Light

35. Heli – Sun Ray
36. Helmi – Pearl
37. Henrik – Home Ruler
38. Iida – Work
39. Iiro – Watchful, Vigilant
40. Ilari – Cheerful, Happy
41. Ilona – Joy
42. Ilta – Evening
43. Inari – Lake
44. Inka – Hero's Daughter
45. Ismo – Devoted to God
46. Jaakko – Supplanter
47. Jalmari – Helmeted Warrior
48. Jari – Helmeted Warrior
49. Jere – God will Uplift
50. Jorma – Farmer
51. Juhani – God is Gracious
52. Juho – God will Add
53. Jukka – God is Gracious
54. Kaarina – Pure
55. Kai – Rejoice
56. Kaisa – Pure
57. Kalle – Free Man
58. Kari – Gust of Wind
59. Katja – Pure
60. Kerttu – Bird
61. Kirsi – Christian
62. Kuisma – Beauty, Order
63. Lari – Laurel
64. Laura – Laurel
65. Leena – Light
66. Leevi – Joined in Harmony
67. Lempi – Love
68. Liisa – God is my Oath
69. Lotta – Free Woman
70. Maarit – Pearl

71. Maikki – Who is Like God?
72. Malla – Strong in War
73. Markku – Warlike
74. Martti – Warlike
75. Matias – Gift of God
76. Meri – The Sea
77. Mika – Who is Like God?
78. Miina – Love
79. Mirja – Wished-for Child
80. Nelli – Shining Light
81. Niilo – People's Victory
82. Oiva – Excellent
83. Olavi – Ancestor's Descendant
84. Onni – Happiness, Luck
85. Orvo – Stranger, Foreigner
86. Oskari – God's Spear
87. Otso – Bear
88. Paavo – Small
89. Pekka – Stone
90. Pentti – Blessed
91. Pirkko – Bright, Shining
92. Raimo – Protecting Hands
93. Risto – Follower of Christ
94. Saku – Remembered by God
95. Seppo – Smith
96. Taina – Secret
97. Tapani – Crown
98. Tarja – Instigator
99. Tuomas – Twin
100. Veikko – Brother

Greek baby names and their meanings

1. Achilles – The hero of the Trojan War
2. Adonis – Lord
3. Agatha – Good-hearted
4. Agnes – Pure or holy
5. Alexander – Defender of mankind
6. Althea – Healer
7. Anastasia – Resurrection
8. Andrew – Manly
9. Angela – Messenger of God
10. Anthony – Priceless one
11. Ariadne – Very holy
12. Artemis – Goddess of the hunt
13. Athena – Goddess of wisdom and warfare
14. Basil – Royal
15. Calliope – Beautiful voice
16. Cassandra – She who entangles men
17. Catherine – Pure
18. Clio – Proclaimer
19. Constantine – Steadfast
20. Cosmo – Order
21. Cyrus – Far sighted
22. Damon – Constant, loyal
23. Danae – Parched
24. Daphne – Laurel tree
25. Demetrius – Devoted to Demeter
26. Diana – Divine
27. Dion – Child of heaven and earth
28. Eirene – Peace
29. Elektra – Shining, bright
30. Elias – The Lord is my God
31. Eros – Love
32. Eugene – Well-born, noble
33. Eulalia – Sweet-speaking
34. Eunice – Good victory

35. Evangeline – Good news
36. Felix – Happy, fortunate
37. Galen – Calm
38. George – Farmer
39. Gregory – Watchful, alert
40. Helen – Bright, shining one
41. Hermione – Messenger
42. Hestia – Goddess of the hearth
43. Hyacinth – Flower
44. Irene – Peace
45. Iris – Rainbow
46. Isidore – Gift of Isis
47. Jason – Healer
48. Jerome – Sacred name
49. Joanna – God is gracious
50. Julia – Youthful
51. Kassandra – She who entangles men
52. Kostas – Constant, steadfast
53. Kyra – Lady
54. Leo – Lion
55. Leonidas – Lion's son
56. Lydia – Woman from Lydia
57. Magdalene – Woman from Magdala
58. Melinda – Honey
59. Melissa – Honey bee
60. Michael – Who is like God?
61. Myron – Sweet oil, perfume
62. Nectar – Drink of the gods
63. Nicholas – Victory of the people
64. Olympia – From Olympus
65. Ophelia – Help
66. Orion – Rising in the sky
67. Pandora – All gifted
68. Paris – Lover
69. Penelope – Weaver
70. Persephone – Bringer of destruction

71. Peter – Stone, rock
72. Phoebe – Bright, pure
73. Phyllis – Leafy foliage
74. Rhea – Flowing stream
75. Selene – Moon
76. Sophia – Wisdom
77. Soteria – Salvation
78. Stavros – Cross
79. Stella – Star
80. Stephen – Crown
81. Thalia – To flourish
82. Thea – Goddess
83. Theodore – Gift of God
84. Theodosia – God's gift
85. Theophilus – Friend of God
86. Theresa – Summer, harvest
87. Theron – Hunter
88. Thomas – Twin
89. Timothy – Honoring God
90. Titus – Honorable
91. Urania – Heavenly
92. Valeria – Strength, health
93. Xenia – Hospitality
94. Yanni – God is gracious
95. Zephyr – West wind
96. Zoe – Life
97. Zosma – Girdle
98. Eudora – Good gift
99. Leander – Lion man
100. Lysandra – Liberator

Turkish baby names and their meanings

1. Ada - Island
2. Adem - Earth
3. Alev - Flame
4. Altan - Red dawn
5. Aras - Plain
6. Arda - He who comes from the field
7. Aslı - Genuine, original
8. Ayberk - Bright moon
9. Aydın - Enlightened
10. Aylin - Moon halo
11. Ayşe - Alive, she who lives
12. Bahar - Spring
13. Barış - Peace
14. Başak - Wheat, Virgo
15. Batu - Firm, strong
16. Beril - Shining sea
17. Berke - Hard, tough
18. Bora - Storm, squall
19. Burak - Bright, shining
20. Can - Life, soul
21. Cem - Ruler, king
22. Ceren - Baby gazelle
23. Ceylan - Gazelle
24. Cihan - Universe, cosmos
25. Damla - Drop
26. Deniz - Sea
27. Derin - Deep
28. Devrim - Revolution
29. Dilara - She who delights the heart
30. Dilek - Wish, desire
31. Doruk - Mountain top
32. Duygu - Emotion, feeling
33. Ediz - High, lofty
34. Ege - Aegean

35. Ekin - Harvest
36. Elif - Slim, tall
37. Emel - Desire, hope
38. Emir - Prince, commander
39. Emre - Brother, friend
40. Enes - Human being
41. Eren - Saint
42. Erol - Brave, heroic
43. Esra - Night journey
44. Evren - Universe, cosmos
45. Ezgi - Melody
46. Fırat - Euphrates River
47. Gamze - Dimple
48. Gizem - Mystery
49. Gökhan - Sky lord
50. Gül - Rose
51. Hakan - Emperor, ruler
52. Hale - Halo around the moon
53. Hande - Smiling, laughing
54. Harun - Aaron
55. Hatice - Early born
56. Işık - Light
57. İlker - First man
58. İpek - Silk
59. Kaan - Prince, lord
60. Kaya - Rock
61. Leyla - Night
62. Melis - Honey bee
63. Mert - Brave, gallant
64. Miray - Moon water
65. Nazlı - Delicate, gentle
66. Onur - Honor, pride
67. Orhan - Great leader
68. Ömer - Long-lived
69. Özge - Different, distinctive
70. Pelin - Wormwood plant

71. Rüzgar - Wind
72. Selin - Flowing water
73. Semih - Generous
74. Seren - Baby gazelle
75. Sinem - My heart, my love
76. Taha - Pure, innocent
77. Talha - A kind of tree
78. Taner - Dawn man
79. Tuna - Danube River
80. Umut - Hope
81. Yağmur - Rain
82. Yavuz - Resolute, stern
83. Yiğit - Brave, valiant
84. Zeynep - Father's precious jewel
85. Ziya - Light, splendor
86. Canan - Beloved
87. Cenk - Battle, war
88. Cemre - Ember
89. Derya - Sea
90. Ebru - Marbled paper art
91. Elvan - Colors
92. Emine - Trustworthy
93. Feride - Unique, singular
94. Gökçe - Sky blue
95. İlhan - Prince, emperor
96. Kerem - Noble, generous
97. Merve - A mountain in paradise
98. Nil - Nile River
99. Öykü - Story, tale
100. Sema - Sky

Egyptian baby names and their meanings

1. Aisha - Living, prosperous
2. Amun - Hidden one
3. Anubis - Royal child
4. Asim - Protector
5. Aziza - Precious
6. Badru - Born during a full moon
7. Basim - Smiling
8. Cairo - Victorious
9. Dalilah - Guide
10. Dua - Worship
11. Ebonee - Black
12. Fahim - Understanding
13. Farida - Unique
14. Gamal - Beauty
15. Haji - Born during the Hajj
16. Hasina - Good
17. Heba - Gift from God
18. Isis - Throne
19. Jamila - Beautiful
20. Kamilah - Perfect
21. Khepri - Morning sun
22. Layla - Night
23. Maat - Truth
24. Menna - Destiny
25. Nefertari - Beautiful companion
26. Osiris - Powerful
27. Qabil - Able
28. Ra - Sun
29. Sabah - Morning
30. Tahira - Pure
31. Umm - Mother
32. Zahi - Bright
33. Zuberi - Strong
34. Aida - Returner

35. Akil - Intelligent
36. Bahiti - Fortune
37. Cleopatra - Glory of the father
38. Dendera - From Dendera
39. Eshe - Life
40. Femi - Love me
41. Gahiji - Hunter
42. Habibah - Beloved
43. Imhotep - Peace
44. Jabari - Brave
45. Kahlil - Friend
46. Lateef - Gentle
47. Mafuane - Earth
48. Nia - Purpose
49. Omari - God the highest
50. Ptah - Creator
51. Rashidi - Wise
52. Safiya - Pure
53. Tahir - Pure
54. Umi - Life
55. Zahra - Flower
56. Zuri - Beautiful
57. Adio - Righteous
58. Amenhotep - Peace of Amun
59. Bastet - She of the ointment jar
60. Dalia - Grapevine
61. Edfu - From Edfu
62. Fadil - Generous
63. Giza - From Giza
64. Halima - Gentle
65. Isha - Alive
66. Jamil - Handsome
67. Khepri - Morning sun
68. Latif - Kind
69. Mena - Eternal
70. Nefertiti - The beautiful one has come

71. Oba - King
72. Qadim - Ancient
73. Ramesses - Born of Ra
74. Sekhmet - Powerful
75. Tia - Princess
76. Uraeus - Sacred serpent
77. Zaliki - Well-born
78. Zuka - Free
79. Akila - Intelligent
80. Amunet - The hidden one
81. Bakt - Servant
82. Cleon - Famous
83. Duat - Underworld
84. Esna - From Esna
85. Fathi - Conqueror
86. Gamil - Handsome
87. Hapi - God of the Nile
88. Isi - Deer
89. Jomana - Pearl
90. Keket - Goddess of darkness
91. Lapis - Stone
92. Mansa - King
93. Nour - Light
94. Osaze - God chooses
95. Qaletaqa - Guardian of the people
96. Rami - Archer
97. Sadeek - Friend
98. Tawfiq - Success
99. Uzuri - Beauty
100. Zesiro - First born of twins

South African baby names and their meanings

1. Aaliyah – Highly exalted
2. Abri – Mother of many nations
3. Ayanda – They augment
4. Amahle – The beautiful ones
5. Buhle – Beauty
6. Bandile – They have multiplied and grown
7. Cebile – Rich in possessions
8. Dakalo – Happiness
9. Enzokuhle – Do good
10. Fikile – She has arrived
11. Gugu – Precious
12. Hlengiwe – Rescued
13. Inathi – God is with us
14. Jabulile – Be happy
15. Khanyi – Light
16. Lethabo – Joy
17. Mbalenhle – Beautiful flower
18. Nandi – Sweet
19. Olwethu – Our own
20. Palesa – Flower
21. Qhawe – Hero
22. Rethabile – We are happy
23. Siphesihle – Beautiful gift
24. Thando – Love
25. Uyanda – She is growing
26. Vuyiswa – To be visited
27. Wethu – Ours
28. Xolani – Peace
29. Yoliswa – To be visited
30. Zinhle – The beautiful ones
31. Afrika – After the continent
32. Bhekizizwe – Look after the nations
33. Cyprian – From Cyprus

34. Dumi – Fame
35. Esihle – Beautiful
36. Fana – He appears
37. Gcinumuzi – Keep the heritage
38. Hlompho – Respect
39. Itumeleng – Joy
40. Jabu – Joy
41. Khaya – Home
42. Lindo – Wait
43. Mpho – Gift
44. Nkosi – Lord
45. Onke – All
46. Phiwokuhle – Gift
47. Qaqamba – Bright, shining
48. Rorisang – Praise
49. Sfiso – Light
50. Thabo – Joy
51. Unathi – God is with us
52. Vuyo – Joy
53. Wandile – They have multiplied
54. Xola – Stay in peace
55. Yonela – Enough
56. Zola – Tranquil
57. Andile – They have multiplied
58. Bongani – Be thankful
59. Celiwe – The one who has been crowned
60. Dumisani – Praise
61. Enhle – Beautiful
62. Fikani – Think
63. Gugulethu – Our precious one
64. Hlonipha – Respect
65. Inam – God is with us
66. Jabulani – Be happy
67. Khulani – Grow
68. Lindani – Wait
69. Muzi – Home

70. Nkosinathi – God is with us
71. Oupa – Grandfather
72. Phumzile – Rest
73. Qondile – Calm
74. Rethabile – We are happy
75. Sipho – Gift
76. Thulani – Be quiet
77. Uzile – Glory
78. Vusumuzi – Rekindle the family
79. Wandisile – They have increased
80. Xolile – Forgiven
81. Yanga – Prosper
82. Zanele – They are enough
83. Andiswa – Increase
84. Bonginkosi – Thank the Lord
85. Celiwe – Crowned
86. Dumisa – Praise
87. Entle – Beauty
88. Funani – Search
89. Gcina – Keep
90. Hlubi – Good
91. Iniko – Born during troubled times
92. Jabu – Joy
93. Khumo – Wealth
94. Lindiwe – Waited for
95. Mthunzi – Shade
96. Nkanyezi – Star
97. Olwethu – It's ours
98. Phindile – You have found
99. Qhama – Bright
100. Radebe – We have given

Nigerian baby names and their meanings

1. Abiodun - Born during a festival
2. Adanna - Father's daughter
3. Ademola - Crown brings happiness
4. Afolabi - Born into high status
5. Aisha - Life
6. Akachi - Hand of God
7. Akin - Brave
8. Amara - Grace
9. Babatunde - Father has returned
10. Bolanle - Finds wealth at home
11. Chidi - God exists
12. Chijindu - God holds life
13. Chika - God is supreme
14. Chinua - God's own blessing
15. Chinyere - God gave
16. Chizoba - God protect us
17. Dapo - Born with wealth
18. Durosinmi - Wait and rest in wealth
19. Ebun - Gift
20. Efe - Wealth
21. Efosa - Wealth from God
22. Emeka - God has done great
23. Eniola - Wealthy person
24. Eze - King
25. Femi - Love me
26. Funke - Given to God
27. Gbenga - Lift up
28. Ife - Love
29. Ifeoluwa - Love of God
30. Ijeoma - Safe journey
31. Ikechukwu - Power of God
32. Ireti - Hope
33. Jadesola - Come into wealth
34. Jumoke - Everyone loves the child

35. Kehinde - The second-born of twins
36. Kola - Bring in wealth
37. Kunle - Filled our home with wealth
38. Morenike - I have someone to cherish
39. Ngozi - Blessing
40. Nkem - My own
41. Obi - Heart
42. Obioma - Kind heart
43. Odunayo - Year of joy
44. Okeke - Born on market day
45. Olabisi - Joy is multiplied
46. Olajide - Wealth awakes
47. Olamide - My wealth has come
48. Olanrewaju - Wealth is moving forward
49. Olasunkanmi - Wealth moves closer to me
50. Oluchi - God's work
51. Olufemi - God loves me
52. Olumide - God has arrived
53. Olusegun - God is victorious
54. Oluwakemi - God cherishes me
55. Oluwatobi - God is great
56. Onyeka - Who is greater than God
57. Onyekachi - Who is greater than God
58. Opeyemi - I give thanks
59. Orji - Tree of life
60. Osasere - God makes perfection
61. Seyi - This one is precious
62. Simisola - Rest in wealth
63. Taiwo - Taste the world
64. Temitope - Enough to give thanks
65. Toluwalope - God's worth of praise
66. Uche - Thought, mind
67. Uchenna - God's will
68. Ugochi - God's glory
69. Uzoma - Good journey
70. Wale - To arrive home

71. Yemi - Befitting me
72. Yewande - Mother has returned
73. Zainab - Beautiful, precious
74. Zikora - Show the world
75. Adebayo - The crown meets joy
76. Adetokunbo - The crown came from over the sea
77. Akinlabi - We have a boy
78. Ayotunde - Joy has returned
79. Chibuzo - God leads
80. Chidiebere - God is merciful
81. Chidubem - God is my guide
82. Chinedu - God leads
83. Chukwudi - God exists
84. Ekenedilichukwu - Thanks be to God
85. Ifechukwude - What God has written
86. Iheanacho - What we are looking for
87. Ihechiluru - Light of God
88. Ikechukwukwu - Power of God
89. Kelechukwu - Thank God
90. Nnamdi - My father is alive
91. Obinna - Father's heart
92. Okechukwu - God's portion
93. Okwukwe - Faith
94. Olufunmilayo - God gave me joy
95. Olumuyiwa - God brought this
96. Onyedikachi - Who is like God
97. Onyemachi - Who knows God's mind
98. Ugochukwukwu - Glory of God
99. Uzochukwu - God's way
100. Yemisi - Honor me

Kenyan baby names and their meanings

1. Adongo – Firstborn of twins
2. Akello – Second born after twins
3. Achieng – Born when the sun is shining
4. Auma – Born during the day
5. Abuya – Born when the garden is overgrown
6. Adhiambo – Born after sunset
7. Anyango – Friend
8. Ayoo – Born on a joyful occasion
9. Bena – You are the next
10. Chacha – Strong
11. Chike – God's power
12. Chege – Small home
13. Daudi – Beloved
14. Esiaka – Born during locust season
15. Esiankiki – Youngest daughter
16. Fadhili – Kindness, generosity
17. Gacoki – Joy
18. Gakere – Small and strong
19. Gitonga – Rich person
20. Habari – News
21. Halima – Gentle, patient
22. Imara – Firm, steadfast
23. Jengo – Building
24. Juma – Born on Friday
25. Kamau – Quiet warrior
26. Kakenya – Active in the morning
27. Kanja – Born during a famine
28. Kioni – Someone who sees
29. Lulu – Precious
30. Lusala – Born during locust season
31. Maalim – Teacher
32. Makena – The happy one
33. Mumbi – Creator
34. Mwaniki – Born during the rainy season

35. Nia – Purpose
36. Njau – Young bull
37. Nyawira – Hardworking
38. Nyokabi – Born during the dry season
39. Okoth – Born when it's raining
40. Omondi – Born early in the morning
41. Onyango – Born early in the morning
42. Pili – Second born
43. Raha – Joy, happiness
44. Rukiya – Ascend, rise
45. Siti – Lady, woman
46. Tumaini – Hope
47. Umi – Life
48. Wairimu – One who loves farming
49. Wanjiru – Daughter of a shepherd
50. Zuri – Beautiful
51. Zawadi – Gift
52. Yaa – Born on Thursday
53. Xola – Stay in peace
54. Wamalwa – Born during the brewing season
55. Wambui – Singer of songs
56. Wacera – The wanderer
57. Wambua – Born during the rainy season
58. Wainaina – Gatherer of firewood
59. Wanyonyi – Born during the weeding season
60. Wamuyu – Daughter of a rich man
61. Wanjala – Born during famine
62. Wanjiku – Daughter of the earth
63. Wanyama – Born during the animal migration season
64. Waruguru – Born after many girls
65. Wacuka – Daughter of a judge
66. Wairiako – Daughter of a storyteller
67. Wamalwa – Born during the brewing season
68. Wanjala – Born during famine

69. Wanyama – Born during the animal migration season
70. Waruguru – Born after many girls
71. Wacuka – Daughter of a judge
72. Wairiako – Daughter of a storyteller
73. Wamuyu – Daughter of a rich man
74. Wanjiku – Daughter of the earth
75. Wanyonyi – Born during the weeding season
76. Wambui – Singer of songs
77. Wacera – The wanderer
78. Wambua – Born during the rainy season
79. Wainaina – Gatherer of firewood
80. Wamalwa – Born during the brewing season
81. Wanjala – Born during famine
82. Wanjiku – Daughter of the earth
83. Wanyama – Born during the animal migration season
84. Waruguru – Born after many girls
85. Wacuka – Daughter of a judge
86. Wairiako – Daughter of a storyteller
87. Wamuyu – Daughter of a rich man
88. Wanjiku – Daughter of the earth
89. Wanyonyi – Born during the weeding season
90. Wambui – Singer of songs
91. Wacera – The wanderer
92. Wambua – Born during the rainy season
93. Wainaina – Gatherer of firewood
94. Wamalwa – Born during the brewing season
95. Wanjala – Born during famine
96. Wanjiku – Daughter of the earth
97. Wanyama – Born during the animal migration season
98. Waruguru – Born after many girls
99. Wacuka – Daughter of a judge
100. Wairiako – Daughter of a storyteller

Ghanaian baby names and their meanings

1. Aba – Born on Thursday
2. Abena – Born on Tuesday
3. Adjoa – Born on Monday
4. Afia – Born on Friday
5. Agyei – God's strength
6. Akua – Born on Wednesday
7. Amma – Born on Saturday
8. Ato – Born on Wednesday
9. Badu – Tenth born child
10. Boahen – Leader or king
11. Boakye – Adventurous
12. Dakari – Happiness
13. Dede – Grasshopper or locust
14. Ebo – Born on Tuesday
15. Efia – Born on Friday
16. Ekua – Born on Wednesday
17. Fynn – White or fair
18. Gyasi – Wonderful
19. Kofi – Born on Friday
20. Kwame – Born on Saturday
21. Kwabena – Born on Tuesday
22. Kwadwo – Born on Monday
23. Kwaku – Born on Wednesday
24. Kweku – Born on Wednesday
25. Kwesi – Born on Sunday
26. Maame – Mother
27. Nana – King or Queen
28. Nyamekye – God's gift
29. Obi – Heart
30. Ohene – King
31. Panyin – Elder twin
32. Sisi – Born on Sunday
33. Yaa – Born on Thursday
34. Yaw – Born on Thursday

35. Abam – Second child after twins
36. Adusa – Thirteenth born
37. Baah – Born on Thursday
38. Esi – Born on Sunday
39. Frempomaa – Noble or respectable woman
40. Kwamina – Born on Saturday
41. Manu – Second born
42. Nhyira – Blessing
43. Nkansah – Ninth born
44. Nyankomago – Seventh born
45. Ofori – Born on Friday
46. Ohemaa – Queen
47. Osei – Noble or honorable
48. Oteng – Born on Wednesday
49. Owusu – Strong-willed or determined
50. Serwaa – Noblewoman
51. Tawiah – First child after twins
52. Yawson – Seventh born
53. Adoma – Beautiful child
54. Akosua – Born on Sunday
55. Ameyaw – Praise to God
56. Boatemaa – Queen mother
57. Danso – Reliable or dependable
58. Eshun – Sixth born
59. Kakra – Second twin
60. Kunto – Third born after twins
61. Nkrumah – Ninth born
62. Oheneba – Prince or princess
63. Opoku – Powerful or strong
64. Poku – Born to a king or queen
65. Sefa – Seventh born
66. Twum – Born after twins
67. Yamoah – God knows
68. Yawo – Born on Thursday
69. Acheampong – Destined for greatness
70. Adjei – Born on Monday

71. Amoako – Great warrior
72. Boadi – Left-handed
73. Duah – Second-born twin
74. Frimpong – Strong or powerful
75. Kyei – Blessed by God
76. Nsiah – Sixth born
77. Obeng – Born after twins
78. Oforiwaa – Born on Friday
79. Osei – Noble or honorable
80. Poku – Born to a king or queen
81. Serwa – Noblewoman
82. Takyi – Blessed by God
83. Yaw – Born on Thursday
84. Yirenkyi – God is watching
85. Adom – Blessing
86. Akoto – Second born after twins
87. Amankwah – Fifth born
88. Boamah – Strong or powerful
89. Dankwa – Fourth born
90. Eno – Fifth born
91. Kyeremeh – Last born
92. Ntim – Eighth born
93. Obiri – Born on Monday
94. Offei – Snake
95. Owusua – Born on Wednesday
96. Prah – Born on a journey
97. Sekyere – Wise or intelligent
98. Tandoh – Third born
99. Yeboah – Left-handed
100. Yentumi – Cannot contest

Ethiopian baby names and their meanings

1. Abeba - Flower
2. Abenet - You are good
3. Addis - New
4. Adanech - She has rescued them
5. Adina - She has saved
6. Afework - Speaks pleasant things
7. Alem - World
8. Alemayehu - I have seen the world
9. Alemitu - She has hidden
10. Amare - Handsome
11. Amari - Handsome
12. Amsalu - Example of the world
13. Assefa - He has increased our joy
14. Aster - Star
15. Ayana - Beautiful flower
16. Bekele - To grow
17. Berhanu - His light
18. Betelhem - House of bread
19. Biruk - Blessed
20. Birtukan - Orange fruit
21. Chaltu - The best
22. Chanyalew - You are my property
23. Dagim - Rainy season
24. Dawit - Beloved
25. Desta - Happiness
26. Eleni - Light
27. Ermias - God has uplifted
28. Eyob - Job, the biblical character
29. Fasil - Castle
30. Fekadu - Seed
31. Fikir - Love
32. Frehiwot - Fruit of life
33. Gedion - Destroyer
34. Genet - Paradise

35. Girma - He is respected
36. Haben - Pride
37. Habtamu - Rich in wisdom
38. Haile - Power
39. Hana - Happiness
40. Hiwot - Life
41. Kalkidan - Promise
42. Kedir - Strong
43. Kifle - My property
44. Kokeb - Star
45. Lelise - She has been heard
46. Lidya - Noble one
47. Mahlet - Harp
48. Mamo - My uncle
49. Mekdes - Temple
50. Mekonnen - The angel
51. Melaku - Angel
52. Meseret - Foundation
53. Mesfin - The end of the mass
54. Mihret - Mercy
55. Mikael - Who is like God
56. Miriam - Biblical name for Mary
57. Nardos - Rose
58. Nebiyu - Prophet
59. Nebiyou - My prophet
60. Negash - King
61. Negussie - My king
62. Rahel - Sheep
63. Rediet - She is accepted
64. Roman - She is incredible
65. Salamawit - She is my peace
66. Samrawit - She is my secret
67. Selam - Peace
68. Selamawit - She is my peace
69. Semira - Fulfilled
70. Senait - They are happy

71. Seble - Harvest
72. Sisay - Increase
73. Sitota - Gift
74. Tadesse - Rebirth
75. Tadewos - Rebirth of God
76. Tamirat - Miracle
77. Tariku - History
78. Teferi - My hope
79. Tewodros - Theodore, gift of God
80. Tigist - Patience
81. Tsedey - My justice
82. Tsion - Zion
83. Wubalem - Beautiful
84. Wubit - Flower
85. Yared - He is afraid
86. Yemisrach - Summer
87. Yeshi - For a thousand
88. Yohannes - John, the biblical character
89. Zebene - My crown
90. Zelalem - Eternal
91. Zemene - My song
92. Zena - News
93. Zerihun - The seed
94. Zewditu - The crown
95. Zinabu - My news
96. Zufan - My precious
97. Zuriash - My gold
98. Zewde - My crown
99. Zelalem - My eternity
100. Zenebe - My man

Moroccan baby names and their meanings

1. Aaliyah - Exalted, sublime
2. Abdellah - Servant of Allah
3. Adil - Just, honest
4. Aicha - Alive
5. Ahmed - Praiseworthy
6. Amal - Hope
7. Amina - Safe, secure
8. Anas - Affection, love
9. Asma - Supreme
10. Bilal - Water, freshness
11. Chaima - With a beauty spot
12. Dounia - The world
13. El Hassan - The good, the handsome
14. Fatima - One who abstains
15. Ghizlan - Gazelle
16. Hakim - Wise, judicious
17. Hana - Happiness, bliss
18. Idriss - Studious
19. Imane - Faith, belief
20. Jamal - Beauty
21. Karim - Generous
22. Khadija - Premature child
23. Laila - Night
24. Malik - King, owner
25. Mariam - Sea of bitterness
26. Mustapha - The chosen one
27. Nadia - Caller, announcer
28. Omar - Life, long living
29. Rachid - Rightly guided
30. Salim - Safe, sound
31. Samira - Companion in evening talk
32. Tariq - Morning star
33. Yasmine - Jasmine flower
34. Zainab - Father's joy

35. Zahir - Shining, radiant
36. Zahra - Flower, blossom
37. Ziad - Growth, abundance
38. Abeer - Fragrance
39. Badr - Full moon
40. Basim - Smiling
41. Dalia - Vine
42. Faisal - Decisive
43. Farida - Unique, matchless
44. Hamza - Lion
45. Isra - Nocturnal journey
46. Jamila - Beautiful
47. Khalid - Eternal
48. Latifa - Gentle, kind
49. Mounir - Shining
50. Naima - Comfort, tranquillity
51. Qasim - One who distributes
52. Rania - Queen
53. Sabir - Patient
54. Tamim - Complete, perfect
55. Wafa - Faithfulness
56. Yasir - Wealthy
57. Zafir - Victorious
58. Zohra - Venus, jewel
59. Fadil - Generous, honorable
60. Inas - Sociability
61. Jawad - Generous
62. Khaled - Immortal
63. Lamia - Brilliant, lustrous
64. Mouna - Wish, desire
65. Najwa - Secret, whisper
66. Qadir - Capable, powerful
67. Rahma - Mercy
68. Saad - Felicity
69. Tahar - Pure, chaste
70. Walid - Newborn

71. Yara - Small butterfly
72. Zaki - Pure
73. Amira - Princess
74. Bahija - Joyful, happy
75. Dalal - Treated or touched in a kind and loving way
76. Fatin - Captivating, alluring
77. Houda - Guidance
78. Ibtisam - Smile
79. Jalal - Majesty, grandeur
80. Kamal - Perfection
81. Layla - Night
82. Mona - Noble, aristocratic
83. Nada - Dew, generosity
84. Qamar - Moon
85. Rabia - Spring, springtime
86. Sana - Brilliance, majesty
87. Taha - Pure
88. Widad - Love, friendship
89. Yaqub - Supplanter
90. Zakaria - God has remembered
91. Amine - Faithful, trustworthy
92. Bouchra - Good news
93. Dounia - The world
94. Fauzi - Victorious
95. Hicham - Generosity
96. Iman - Faith, belief
97. Jalila - Great, revered
98. Karam - Generosity
99. Leila - Night
100. Nabil - Noble, generous

Algerian baby names and their meanings

1. Abdel - servant of God
2. Amina - truthful or trustworthy
3. Amira - princess
4. Badr - full moon
5. Bahija - joyful or happy
6. Bilal - water
7. Chaima - with a beauty spot
8. Dalila - guide
9. Elina - intelligent
10. Fadil - generous or noble
11. Fakhri - honorary
12. Farida - unique or precious
13. Ghazi - warrior
14. Hafsa - lioness
15. Hakim - wise
16. Idris - interpreter or studious
17. Iman - faith
18. Jamal - beauty
19. Jamila - beautiful
20. Karim - generous
21. Khalil - friend
22. Lina - tender or compassionate
23. Malik - king
24. Malika - queen
25. Mansour - victorious
26. Mouna - desire or wish
27. Nadia - hope
28. Nafisa - precious
29. Najwa - secret conversation
30. Omar - flourishing or long-lived
31. Rabia - springtime
32. Rafiq - friend
33. Rahim - merciful
34. Rania - queen

35. Rashid - guided one
36. Rayan - watered or luxuriant
37. Sabir - patient
38. Salim - safe or sound
39. Samir - entertaining companion
40. Sana - brilliance or to gaze
41. Sofiane - devoted
42. Tariq - morning star
43. Yasmin - jasmine flower
44. Zahra - flower or blossom
45. Zainab - father's jewel
46. Zaki - pure
47. Zohra - blossom
48. Fathi - conqueror
49. Louna - moon
50. Amine - faithful
51. Hana - happiness
52. Ayoub - repentant
53. Leila - night
54. Youssef - God will increase
55. Kamil - perfect
56. Basma - smile
57. Ilyas - the lord is my God
58. Noor - light
59. Aya - miracle
60. Adam - man
61. Sara - princess
62. Ali - exalted
63. Salma - safe
64. Fatima - captivating
65. Anis - friendly
66. Meryem - beloved
67. Hamza - strong
68. Selma - peace
69. Imran - exalted nation
70. Aicha - alive

71. Amal - hope
72. Dounia - worldly life
73. Samia - elevated
74. Hassan - handsome
75. Sofia - wisdom
76. Ahmed - praiseworthy
77. Layla - night
78. Nour - light
79. Mohamed - praiseworthy
80. Kenza - treasure
81. Ibrahim - father of many
82. Nesrine - wild rose
83. Mehdi - guided one
84. Yasmine - jasmine flower
85. Samira - companion in evening talk
86. Yacine - wealthy
87. Hiba - gift from God
88. Ismail - God will hear
89. Rym - gazelle
90. Amira - princess
91. Nabil - noble
92. Ines - pure
93. Aymen - lucky
94. Lamia - shining
95. Walid - newborn
96. Saida - happy
97. Ayman - blessed
98. Rania - queen
99. Zinedine - beauty of the faith
100. Khaled - eternal

Tunisian baby names and their meanings

1. Aaliyah – Exalted, high
2. Abir – Fragrance
3. Adel – Fair, honest
4. Afif – Chaste, modest
5. Ahlam – Dreams
6. Alia – Noble, high
7. Amal – Hope
8. Amira – Princess
9. Anis – Friendly, companion
10. Asma – Exalted
11. Aya – Miracle
12. Aziz – Powerful, beloved
13. Badr – Full moon
14. Bahija – Joyful, happy
15. Basim – Smiling
16. Bilal – Water, freshness
17. Chaima – With beauty spot
18. Dalia – Grapevine
19. Dalila – Guide, model
20. Dounia – The world
21. Elham – Inspiration
22. Emna – Faithful, to believe
23. Fadil – Generous, honorable
24. Fahd – Panther
25. Farah – Joy, happiness
26. Farid – Unique, precious
27. Fatima – One who abstains
28. Fathi – Conqueror
29. Fida – Redemption, sacrifice
30. Ghada – Graceful, young girl
31. Habib – Beloved
32. Hafsa – Young lioness
33. Hakim – Wise, judicious
34. Halima – Gentle, patient

35. Hamza – Strong, steadfast
36. Hanan – Mercy, compassion
37. Hani – Happy, delighted
38. Hiba – Gift
39. Houda – Right guidance
40. Ibtisam – Smile
41. Idris – Studious, knowledgeable
42. Ikram – Honor, hospitality
43. Ilham – Inspiration
44. Imen – Faith, belief
45. Ismail – God will hear
46. Jamila – Beautiful
47. Jannah – Paradise, garden
48. Jihad – Struggle, holy war
49. Karim – Generous, noble
50. Khalil – Close friend
51. Khadija – Premature child
52. Laila – Night
53. Lamia – Shining, radiant
54. Latifa – Gentle, kind
55. Leila – Night
56. Lina – Palm tree
57. Malik – King, owner
58. Malika – Queen
59. Marwa – Fragrant plant
60. Maryam – Mother of Jesus
61. Mona – Wish, desire
62. Mounir – Shining, luminous
63. Nadia – Caller, announcer
64. Najwa – Secret, whisper
65. Nizar – Little
66. Noor – Light
67. Noura – Light
68. Omar – Long-lived
69. Rabia – Spring
70. Radwan – Pleasure, satisfaction

71. Raja – Hope
72. Ramzi – Symbolic
73. Rashid – Rightly guided
74. Rayan – Luxuriant, plentiful
75. Riad – Gardens
76. Rym – Gazelle
77. Saber – Patient
78. Sabri – Patient
79. Safa – Pure
80. Salim – Safe, sound
81. Sami – High, exalted
82. Samira – Companion in evening conversation
83. Selma – Peace
84. Sofiane – Pure
85. Souad – Happiness, luck
86. Taha – Pure
87. Tahar – Pure, virtuous
88. Tariq – Morning star
89. Walid – Newborn
90. Widad – Love, friendship
91. Yasmine – Jasmine
92. Youssef – God will increase
93. Zainab – Fragrant plant
94. Zaki – Pure
95. Ziad – Abundance
96. Zineb – Beautiful
97. Ziyad – Growth, progress
98. Zohra – Blooming, shining
99. Zouhair – Little flower
100. Zuhra – Venus, brilliance

Libyan baby names and their meanings

1. Aaliyah – High, exalted
2. Aban – Clear, lucid
3. Adnan – Settler
4. Amal – Hope
5. Amani – Wishes, aspirations
6. Amira – Princess
7. Anwar – Light
8. Asim – Protector
9. Ayman – Blessed, lucky
10. Aziza – Precious, cherished
11. Badr – Full moon
12. Bahij – Joyful, happy
13. Basim – Smiling
14. Batul – Ascetic virgin
15. Bilal – Water, freshness
16. Dalia – Vine
17. Dima – Downpour
18. Duha – Morning
19. Farid – Unique, singular
20. Fathi – Conqueror
21. Fatima – Daughter of the Prophet
22. Ghada – Graceful, young girl
23. Habib – Beloved
24. Hadi – Guide
25. Hafsa – Young lioness
26. Hakim – Wise, judicious
27. Halima – Gentle, patient
28. Hamza – Lion
29. Hanan – Compassion, tenderness
30. Hassan – Handsome
31. Huda – Guidance
32. Ibrahim – Father of a multitude
33. Idris – Studious, knowledgeable
34. Ikram – Honor, hospitality

35. Imad – Pillar, support
36. Isra – Night journey
37. Jamal – Beauty
38. Jamila – Beautiful
39. Jawad – Generous
40. Jibril – Angel Gabriel
41. Karam – Generosity
42. Karim – Generous, noble
43. Khalid – Eternal
44. Khadija – Early baby
45. Layla – Night
46. Leila – Night
47. Lina – Palm tree
48. Malik – King
49. Mariam – Bitter
50. Marwan – Solid, quartz
51. Mona – Wishes, desires
52. Nabil – Noble, generous
53. Nadia – Caller
54. Najwa – Secret conversation
55. Nizar – Little
56. Noor – Light
57. Omar – Life, long living
58. Qasim – Divider
59. Rabia – Fourth
60. Radwan – Pleasure, satisfaction
61. Rafiq – Friend
62. Rania – Queen
63. Rashid – Rightly guided
64. Rida – Contentment
65. Sabah – Morning
66. Sabir – Patient
67. Sadik – Truthful
68. Safa – Purity, clarity
69. Safiyya – Pure
70. Sahar – Dawn

71. Salah – Righteousness
72. Salim – Safe, sound
73. Sami – Elevated, sublime
74. Samira – Companion in evening conversation
75. Sara – Princess
76. Selma – Peace
77. Shadi – Singer
78. Suhail – Canopus star
79. Taha – A name of the Prophet Muhammad
80. Tariq – Morning star
81. Thana – Praise
82. Umar – Life, long living
83. Wafa – Loyalty
84. Walid – Newborn
85. Yasir – Wealthy
86. Yasmin – Jasmine flower
87. Youssef – God will increase
88. Zahra – Flower, beauty
89. Zainab – Father's jewel
90. Zaki – Pure
91. Ziyad – Growth, abundance
92. Zuhair – Little flower
93. Zain – Beauty, grace
94. Nizar – Little
95. Tariq – Morning star
96. Yasin – The two
97. Iman – Faith, belief
98. Aisha – Alive, well
99. Faisal – Decisive
100. Hana – Happiness, bliss

Saudi Arabian baby names and their meanings

1. Abdullah - Servant of God
2. Aamir - Prosperous, Civilized
3. Abdulaziz - Servant of the Almighty
4. Adnan - Settler, Resident
5. Ahmed - Much Praised
6. Ali - Exalted, Noble
7. Ammar - Long-Lived
8. Anas - Affection, Love
9. Ayman - Lucky, Righteous
10. Bashar - Bringer of Good News
11. Bilal - The Chosen One
12. Faisal - Judge, Decisive
13. Fahd - Panther, Leopard
14. Faris - Horseman, Knight
15. Ghazi - Warrior, Conqueror
16. Hamza - Strong, Steadfast
17. Hasan - Handsome, Good
18. Hussain - Handsome, Beautiful
19. Ibrahim - Father of Many
20. Idris - Interpreter
21. Imran - Prosperity, Happiness
22. Ismail - God will Hear
23. Jamal - Beauty, Grace
24. Khaled - Eternal, Immortal
25. Malik - King, Owner
26. Mohammed - Praised, Commendable
27. Musa - Saved from the Water
28. Nasser - Helper, Supporter
29. Omar - Long Life, Flourishing
30. Qasim - Distributor, Divider
31. Rashid - Rightly Guided
32. Saad - Good Luck, Good Fortune
33. Salman - Safe, Whole

34. Tariq - Morning Star
35. Yasser - Easy, Wealthy
36. Zaid - Abundance, Growth
37. Zain - Grace, Beauty
38. Aisha - Living, Prosperous
39. Amira - Princess, Leader
40. Fatima - Captivating, Daughter of the Prophet
41. Hana - Happiness, Bliss
42. Huda - Right Guidance
43. Khadija - Premature Child
44. Layla - Night, Born at Night
45. Mariam - Sea of Bitterness, Rebellion
46. Nadia - Caller, Announcer
47. Noor - Light, Brightness
48. Rabia - Spring, Fourth
49. Safiya - Pure, Best Friend
50. Samira - Companion in Evening Talk
51. Yasmin - Jasmine Flower
52. Zahra - Bright, Shining
53. Afnan - Full spreading branches of trees
54. Bader - Full Moon
55. Dalia - Grape vine
56. Eman - Faith
57. Farah - Joy, Happiness
58. Ghada - Graceful woman
59. Hala - Halo around the moon
60. Iman - Faith, Belief
61. Jana - Harvest
62. Kamilah - Perfect
63. Lina - Palm Tree
64. Maha - Wild Cow (Gazelle)
65. Nada - Generosity, Dew
66. Omaima - Little Mother
67. Qamar - Moon
68. Rania - Gazing upon
69. Saba - Morning

70. Tahira - Pure, Clean
71. Umaima - Little Mother
72. Wafa - Loyalty
73. Yara - Small Butterfly
74. Zaina - Beautiful
75. Amal - Hope, Aspiration
76. Buthaina - Gentle, Soft
77. Dunya - World, Universe
78. Fatin - Captivating, Alluring
79. Ghaliya - Fragrant
80. Hiba - Gift
81. Inas - Friendliness, Sociability
82. Jalila - Great, Revered
83. Kamila - Perfect, Complete
84. Lamia - Lustrous, Shining
85. Muna - Wish, Desire
86. Naima - Comfort, Tranquility
87. Oraib - Sharp-minded
88. Qadira - Powerful, Capable
89. Rasha - Young Gazelle
90. Sabah - Morning
91. Tahani - Congratulations
92. Umayma - Little Mother
93. Widad - Love, Friendship
94. Yasmine - Jasmine Flower
95. Zara - Blooming Flower
96. Amna - Peace, Security
97. Bushra - Good News, Glad Tidings
98. Dalal - Treated or Touched in a Kind and Loving Way
99. Fadwa - Sacrificing
100. Ghada - Delicate Young Girl

Iranian baby names and their meanings

1. Aban - Old Arabic name
2. Adel - Just
3. Afsaneh - A fairy tale
4. Ahmad - Much praised
5. Ali - Exalted
6. Alborz - The highest one
7. Amir - Prince
8. Anahita - Immaculate
9. Arash - Bright arrow
10. Arman - Hope
11. Arya - Noble
12. Ashkan - Name of a dynasty
13. Azar - Fire
14. Babak - Little father
15. Bahar - Spring
16. Bahram - Victorious
17. Banu - Lady
18. Behnam - Reputable
19. Behzad - Well-born
20. Bijan - Hero
21. Cyrus - Sun
22. Dara - Wealthy
23. Darius - Preserver
24. Delara - Adorning the heart
25. Ehsan - Charity
26. Elham - Inspiration
27. Farhad - Happiness
28. Farzaneh - Wise
29. Fereshteh - Angel
30. Giti - World
31. Golnar - Flower of Pomegranate
32. Hamid - Praised
33. Hasan - Handsome
34. Hoda - Guidance

35. Iman - Faith
36. Jaleh - Dew
37. Jamal - Beauty
38. Kamran - Successful
39. Kaveh - Ancient hero
40. Kayvan - Saturn
41. Kourosh - Like the sun
42. Laleh - Tulip
43. Layla - Night
44. Leila - Night
45. Mahdi - Guided one
46. Mahnaz - Moon's glory
47. Majid - Glorious
48. Mani - A painter who later claimed to be a prophet
49. Marjan - Coral
50. Maryam - Bitter
51. Masoud - Lucky
52. Mehrdad - Gift of the sun
53. Mitra - Sun
54. Mohammad - Praised one
55. Morteza - Chosen one
56. Nader - Rare
57. Nahid - Immaculate
58. Narges - Narcissus flower
59. Nasrin - Wild rose
60. Navid - Good news
61. Nazanin - Sweetheart
62. Nima - Fair, just
63. Omid - Hope
64. Parisa - Like a fairy
65. Parvin - Pleiades
66. Pedram - Successful
67. Pouriya - A wish
68. Rahim - Merciful
69. Ramin - Joyful
70. Rashid - Rightly guided

71. Reza - Contentment
72. Roshan - Bright
73. Roxana - Dawn
74. Roya - Vision, dream
75. Ruzbeh - Fortunate
76. Saeed - Happy
77. Saman - Jasmine
78. Sara - Pure, happy
79. Shadi - Happiness
80. Shahin - Falcon
81. Shahram - King's fame
82. Shahrzad - City-born
83. Shapour - King's son
84. Simin - Silvery
85. Sohrab - Illustrious, shining
86. Soraya - Pleiades
87. Tahmineh - Strong
88. Tara - Star
89. Vahid - Unique
90. Yasamin - Jasmine
91. Yasmin - Jasmine
92. Yasmine - Jasmine
93. Zahra - Flower
94. Zal - Old
95. Zarina - Golden
96. Ziba - Beautiful
97. Zohreh - Venus
98. Zoya - Alive
99. Zulaikha - Brilliant beauty
100. Zohre - Venus

Iraqi baby names and their meanings

1. Abeer - Fragrance
2. Adnan - Settler
3. Amal - Hope
4. Amani - Wishes
5. Anwar - Light
6. Asif - Gather
7. Aziz - Powerful, Beloved
8. Bahira - Brilliant, Bright
9. Basim - Smiling
10. Bilal - Water, Moisture
11. Dalia - Vine
12. Eman - Faith
13. Fadi - Redeemer
14. Farah - Joy, Happiness
15. Farid - Unique
16. Fawzi - Victorious
17. Ghada - Graceful
18. Hadi - Guide
19. Hala - Halo around the moon
20. Hamza - Lion
21. Hanan - Mercy
22. Hassan - Handsome
23. Haytham - Young eagle
24. Ibtisam - Smile
25. Iman - Faith, Belief
26. Isra - Night Journey
27. Jamal - Beauty
28. Jamila - Beautiful
29. Jawad - Generous
30. Kamil - Perfect
31. Kareem - Noble, Generous
32. Khalid - Eternal
33. Khayri - Charitable
34. Layla - Night

35. Lina - Palm tree
36. Majid - Noble
37. Malik - King
38. Mariam - Sea of bitterness
39. Maysa - To walk with a proud, swinging gait
40. Munir - Luminous
41. Nabil - Noble
42. Nadia - Caller
43. Nasir - Helper
44. Nida - Call
45. Nizar - Little
46. Noor - Light
47. Omar - Long-lived
48. Qasim - Divider
49. Rahim - Merciful
50. Rasha - Young gazelle
51. Rashid - Rightly guided
52. Rida - Contentment
53. Sabah - Morning
54. Sabir - Patient
55. Salah - Righteousness
56. Sami - High, Exalted
57. Samira - Companion in evening conversation
58. Sara - Princess
59. Tariq - Morning star
60. Umar - Life
61. Wafa - Faithfulness
62. Yasir - Wealthy
63. Yasmin - Jasmine
64. Youssef - God will increase
65. Zain - Beauty
66. Zara - Blooming flower
67. Ziad - Abundance
68. Ziyad - To increase
69. Aida - Visitor, Return
70. Akeem - Wise

71. Amira - Princess
72. Ayman - Lucky
73. Baraa - Innocence
74. Faisal - Decisive
75. Hafsa - Lioness
76. Idris - Studious
77. Imran - Prosperity
78. Jafar - Stream
79. Kader - Powerful
80. Laila - Night
81. Majed - Glorious
82. Naim - Comfort, Tranquility
83. Nour - Light
84. Qadir - Capable
85. Raed - Leader
86. Safa - Pure
87. Saleh - Righteous
88. Taha - Pure
89. Waleed - Newborn
90. Yara - Small butterfly
91. Zahra - Flower
92. Zeinab - Fragrant flower
93. Ziad - Superabundance
94. Afnan - Tree branches
95. Baha - Beautiful, Magnificent
96. Dalal - Treated or touched in a kind and loving way
97. Essam - Safeguard
98. Fatin - Clever, Smart
99. Ghassan - Youth, Prime of life
100. Huda - Right guidance

Israeli baby names and their meanings

1. Abigail - Father's joy
2. Adina - Gentle
3. Adir - Mighty, powerful
4. Aharon - Exalted, high mountain
5. Ahava - Love
6. Akiva - Protect, shelter
7. Aliza - Joyful
8. Amos - Carried by God
9. Anat - To sing
10. Ari - Lion
11. Ariel - Lion of God
12. Asher - Happy, blessed
13. Avi - My father
14. Avigail - Father's joy
15. Avishai - My father is a gift
16. Aviv - Spring
17. Aviva - Springlike, fresh
18. Avner - Father of light
19. Bar - Son
20. Barak - Blessing
21. Batya - Daughter of God
22. Ben - Son
23. Benjamin - Son of the right hand
24. Carmel - Vineyard
25. Chaim - Life
26. Chana - Grace
27. Dalia - Branch
28. Daniel - God is my judge
29. Daphne - Laurel
30. David - Beloved
31. Dov - Bear
32. Eden - Delight, paradise
33. Efraim - Fruitful
34. Eitan - Strong, enduring

35. Eli - Ascend
36. Eliezer - God is my help
37. Eliana - My God has answered
38. Elie - The Lord is my God
39. Elisha - God is salvation
40. Erez - Cedar tree
41. Ethan - Enduring, strong
42. Gabriel - God is my strength
43. Gavriel - God is my strength
44. Gil - Joy, happiness
45. Hadas - Myrtle tree
46. Hadassah - Myrtle tree
47. Haim - Life
48. Hana - Grace
49. Hannah - Grace
50. Ilan - Tree
51. Isaac - Laughter
52. Isaiah - Salvation of the Lord
53. Ishai - Gift
54. Jacob - Supplanter
55. Jael - Mountain goat
56. Jonah - Dove
57. Jonathan - God has given
58. Joseph - He will add
59. Joshua - God is salvation
60. Judah - Praise
61. Leah - Weary
62. Levi - Joined, attached
63. Lior - My light
64. Liron - My joy
65. Miriam - Sea of bitterness
66. Moriah - God teaches
67. Moshe - Drawn out
68. Naomi - Pleasantness
69. Natan - Given
70. Nathaniel - Gift of God

71. Noah - Rest, comfort
72. Noam - Pleasantness
73. Oded - To restore
74. Omer - Sheaf of wheat
75. Or - Light
76. Ori - My light
77. Rachel - Ewe
78. Rahel - Ewe
79. Reuben - Behold, a son
80. Rivka - To bind
81. Ron - Song, joy
82. Ruth - Companion, friend
83. Samson - Sun
84. Samuel - God has heard
85. Sarah - Princess
86. Shai - Gift
87. Shalom - Peace
88. Shlomo - Peace
89. Shmuel - God has heard
90. Simcha - Joy
91. Tamar - Palm tree
92. Uri - My light
93. Uriel - God is my light
94. Yael - Mountain goat
95. Yair - He will enlighten
96. Yakir - Precious
97. Yarden - To flow down, descend
98. Yehuda - Praised
99. Yitzhak - He will laugh
100. Zev - Wolf

Palestinian baby names and their meanings

1. Abeer - Fragrance
2. Abir - The fragrance of a flower
3. Adnan - Settler
4. Ahlam - Dreams
5. Aida - Returner
6. Aisha - Lively
7. Akram - Generous
8. Ali - Noble, sublime
9. Amal - Hope, expectation
10. Amani - Wishes, aspirations
11. Amira - Princess
12. Anas - Affection, love
13. Arafat - Knowledgeable
14. Asad - Lion
15. Asil - Noble, pure
16. Asma - Supreme
17. Ayah - Miracle, sign
18. Aziz - Powerful, beloved
19. Badr - Full moon
20. Bahaa - Beauty, glory
21. Baha - Splendor
22. Basim - Smiling
23. Basma - A smile
24. Bilal - Water, freshness
25. Bushra - Good news
26. Dalia - Vine
27. Dalal - Treated or touched in a kind and loving way
28. Dana - Pearl
29. Dina - Love
30. Emad - Pillar, support
31. Fadi - Redeemer
32. Fadwa - Sacrifice
33. Fahd - Lynx
34. Fahim - Understanding, wise

35. Farah - Joy
36. Farid - Unique
37. Fatima - One who abstains
38. Fawzi - Successful
39. Fida - Sacrifice
40. Gamal - Beauty
41. Ghada - Graceful woman
42. Ghassan - Youth, prime of life
43. Hadi - Guide to righteousness
44. Hala - Halo
45. Hamza - Lion
46. Hanan - Mercy
47. Hasan - Handsome
48. Hashim - Destroyer of evil
49. Haya - Life
50. Huda - Right guidance
51. Ibtisam - Smile
52. Ihab - Gift
53. Iman - Faith
54. Isra - Nocturnal journey
55. Jamal - Beauty
56. Jamil - Beautiful
57. Jawad - Generous
58. Jihad - Struggle
59. Jumana - Silver pearl
60. Kamil - Perfect
61. Karim - Generous
62. Khalid - Eternal
63. Khadija - Premature child
64. Layla - Night
65. Lina - Tender
66. Lubna - Storax tree
67. Maha - Wild cow
68. Mahdi - Guided to the right path
69. Mahmoud - Praised
70. Majed - Noble

71. Majida - Glorious
72. Malak - Angel
73. Malik - King
74. Mariam - Sea of bitterness
75. Marwan - Solid
76. Mona - Noble, aristocratic
77. Muna - Wish, desire
78. Nabil - Noble
79. Nadia - Caller
80. Nadim - Friend
81. Nael - Winner
82. Naim - Comfort, tranquility
83. Najwa - Secret conversation
84. Nidal - Struggle
85. Nizar - Little
86. Noor - Light
87. Omar - Life
88. Qasim - Divider
89. Raja - Hope
90. Rami - Archer
91. Rashid - Rightly guided
92. Rima - White antelope
93. Salim - Safe, sound
94. Sami - Exalted
95. Samir - Entertaining companion
96. Sana - Brilliance
97. Tariq - Morning star
98. Yara - Small butterfly
99. Yasmin - Jasmine flower
100. Ziad - Abundance

Jordanian baby names and their meanings

1. Aaliyah - Exalted, sublime
2. Abdullah - Servant of God
3. Adil - Just, honest
4. Ahmad - Highly praised
5. Ali - Noble, sublime
6. Amina - Trustworthy, faithful
7. Amira - Princess
8. Ayman - Lucky, on the right
9. Aziz - Powerful, beloved
10. Bahira - Brilliant, bright
11. Bilal - Water, moisture
12. Dalia - Vine, branch
13. Dalal - Touched in a kind and loving way
14. Fadi - Redeemer, savior
15. Faisal - Decisive
16. Fatima - One who abstains
17. Ghada - Graceful woman
18. Hadi - Guide to righteousness
19. Hana - Happiness, bliss
20. Hassan - Handsome, good
21. Huda - Right guidance
22. Iman - Faith, belief
23. Jamal - Beauty
24. Jamila - Beautiful
25. Khaled - Eternal
26. Laila - Night
27. Leena - Tender
28. Malik - King
29. Mariam - Lady, mistress
30. Mona - Desires, wishes
31. Nabil - Noble, generous
32. Nadia - Caller, announcer
33. Omar - Life, long living
34. Qasim - Divider, distributor

35. Rahim - Merciful, compassionate
36. Rania - Gazing upon
37. Rashid - Rightly guided
38. Rayan - Watered, luxuriant
39. Reem - Gazelle
40. Sami - Elevated, sublime
41. Samira - Entertaining companion
42. Sara - Princess
43. Tariq - Morning star
44. Yasmin - Jasmine flower
45. Zain - Beauty, grace
46. Zeina - Beautiful
47. Ziad - Growth, increase
48. Zara - Blooming flower
49. Layla - Night
50. Fahad - Leopard
51. Noor - Light
52. Salma - Peaceful
53. Yara - Small butterfly
54. Farah - Joy, happiness
55. Sana - Brilliance, radiance
56. Hani - Happy, delighted
57. Maha - Wild cow, deer
58. Noura - Light
59. Aisha - Living, prosperous
60. Bilal - Refreshing
61. Salim - Safe, sound
62. Amal - Hope, expectation
63. Fadi - Savior
64. Nada - Generosity, dew
65. Tala - Stalking wolf
66. Ihab - Gift
67. Lina - Palm tree
68. Ayah - Miracle, sign
69. Sufian - Fast-moving, light
70. Hala - Halo around the moon

71. Nidal - Struggle
72. Rami - Archer
73. Safa - Pure
74. Tarek - Morning star
75. Yasmine - Jasmine flower
76. Zaid - Increase, growth
77. Hiba - Gift
78. Kareem - Generous, noble
79. Lama - Darkness of lips
80. Nour - Light
81. Rasha - Young gazelle
82. Sadeem - Mist, fog
83. Tamara - Date palm tree
84. Wafa - Loyalty
85. Yasin - Rich, prosperous
86. Zaina - Beauty, adornment
87. Haniya - Happy, delighted
88. Kamil - Perfect
89. Layan - Softness, gentleness
90. Nisreen - Flower of Sweet Basil
91. Rawan - Flowing water
92. Saif - Sword
93. Taim - Generous
94. Waleed - Newborn
95. Yasir - Wealthy
96. Zara - Blooming flower
97. Heba - Gift
98. Kamal - Perfection
99. Layal - Nights
100. Nizar - Little

Syrian baby names and their meanings

1. Aaliyah - Exalted, high-ranking
2. Abdullah - Servant of God
3. Abir - Fragrance
4. Adnan - Settler
5. Aisha - Lively, life
6. Alina - Noble, kind
7. Amal - Hope, expectation
8. Ameer - Prince, ruler
9. Amira - Princess
10. Anas - Affection, love
11. Aya - Miracle, sign
12. Ayman - Lucky, blessed
13. Bashar - Bringer of good news
14. Basima - Smiling
15. Bilal - Water, freshness
16. Buthayna - Beautiful, delicate
17. Dalia - Grape vine
18. Dima - Rainy cloud
19. Esra - Night journey
20. Farah - Joy, happiness
21. Farid - Unique, precious
22. Fatin - Captivating, alluring
23. Fawzi - Successful
24. Ghada - Graceful, young girl
25. Hadi - Guide to righteousness
26. Hala - Halo around the moon
27. Hamza - Steadfast, strong
28. Hanan - Mercy, compassion
29. Hani - Happy, delighted
30. Hiba - Gift from God
31. Huda - Right guidance
32. Ibrahim - Father of many
33. Iman - Faith, belief
34. Isra - Night journey

35. Jamal - Beauty
36. Jana - Harvest
37. Jawad - Generous
38. Karam - Generosity
39. Karim - Generous, noble
40. Khalid - Eternal, immortal
41. Khadija - Premature child
42. Layla - Night
43. Leena - Tender
44. Lina - Palm tree
45. Lubna - Storax tree
46. Maha - Wild cow, deer
47. Mahir - Skilled
48. Malak - Angel
49. Mariam - Sea of bitterness
50. Marwan - Solid, quartz
51. Maya - Water
52. Miriam - Sea of bitterness
53. Mona - Noble, aristocratic
54. Muhammad - Praiseworthy
55. Nadia - Caller, announcer
56. Naim - Comfort, tranquility
57. Nizar - Little
58. Noor - Light
59. Omar - Long-lived
60. Qasim - Divider, distributor
61. Rami - Archer
62. Rana - Gazing, looking at
63. Rashid - Rightly guided
64. Rawan - Gazing
65. Reem - Gazelle
66. Rida - Contentment
67. Rima - White antelope
68. Saba - Morning
69. Sabah - Morning
70. Sabir - Patient

71. Sadik - Truthful
72. Salim - Safe, undamaged
73. Sami - Elevated, sublime
74. Samir - Entertaining companion
75. Sara - Princess
76. Selma - Peaceful
77. Shadi - Singer
78. Suhail - Canopus star
79. Taha - Pure
80. Tariq - Morning star
81. Thana - Praise
82. Umar - Life, long-lived
83. Wael - Seeker of refuge
84. Wafa - Loyalty
85. Yahya - God is gracious
86. Yasmin - Jasmine flower
87. Youssef - He will add
88. Zain - Beauty, grace
89. Zaina - Beauty, grace
90. Zara - Blooming flower
91. Ziad - Abundance
92. Zoya - Alive
93. Sana - Brilliance, radiance
94. Salwa - Solace, comfort
95. Samara - Guardian, protected by God
96. Nada - Dew, generosity
97. Laila - Night
98. Kamil - Perfect
99. Jamal - Beauty
100. Idris - Studious, learned

Lebanese baby names and their meanings

1. Aaliyah - Exalted, sublime
2. Abbas - Stern, lion
3. Abir - Fragrance
4. Adel - Righteous, fair
5. Adnan - Settler
6. Ahlam - Dreams
7. Ahmed - Highly praised
8. Aida - Reward, present
9. Aisha - Living, prosperous
10. Ali - Noble, sublime
11. Amal - Hope, aspiration
12. Amira - Princess
13. Anwar - Luminous
14. Aya - Miracle
15. Ayman - Lucky, right-handed
16. Aziz - Powerful, beloved
17. Bahaa - Glory, splendor
18. Basim - Smiling
19. Bilal - Water, freshness
20. Boutros - Stone, rock
21. Camil - Perfect
22. Dalal - Pampered
23. Dalia - Grapevine
24. Dany - God is my judge
25. Elias - Jehovah is God
26. Elie - My God is Yahweh
27. Fadi - Redeemer
28. Fadia - Savior
29. Farah - Joy
30. Farid - Unique, precious
31. Fawzi - Victorious
32. Fouad - Heart
33. Ghada - Graceful, young girl
34. Ghassan - Youth, prime of life

35. Habib - Beloved
36. Hadi - Guiding to the right
37. Hala - Halo around the moon
38. Hamza - Steadfast, lion
39. Hanan - Compassion, mercy
40. Hassan - Handsome, good
41. Hiba - Gift from God
42. Hoda - Guidance
43. Hussein - Handsome, beautiful
44. Ibtisam - Smile
45. Iman - Faith, belief
46. Ismail - God will hear
47. Jamal - Beauty
48. Jamil - Beautiful
49. Jana - Harvest, yield
50. Jihad - Struggle, holy war
51. Karim - Generous, noble
52. Khalil - Friend
53. Lama - Darkness of lips
54. Layla - Night
55. Leila - Night
56. Lina - Tender
57. Malik - King
58. Mariam - Bitter, sea of bitterness
59. Marwan - Solid, quartz
60. Maya - Water
61. Maysa - To walk with a proud, swinging gait
62. Mirna - Beloved
63. Mohamed - Praised, commendable
64. Mona - Noble, aristocratic
65. Nadia - Caller
66. Nadim - Friend, companion
67. Naim - Comfort, ease
68. Naji - Safe
69. Nizar - Little
70. Noor - Light

71.	Omar -	Long-lived
72.	Rami -	Archer
73.	Rana -	Gazing, looking at
74.	Rashad -	Rightly guided
75.	Rima -	White antelope
76.	Rola -	Famous in the land
77.	Samir -	Entertaining companion
78.	Sara -	Princess
79.	Selim -	Safe, undamaged
80.	Sema -	Divine omen
81.	Shadi -	Singer
82.	Siham -	Arrows
83.	Tala -	Palm tree
84.	Talal -	Admirable
85.	Tamara -	Date palm
86.	Tarek -	Morning star
87.	Wafa -	Faithfulness
88.	Walid -	Newborn
89.	Yasmin -	Jasmine
90.	Youssef -	God will increase
91.	Zain -	Beauty, grace
92.	Zaina -	Beautiful
93.	Zara -	Blooming flower
94.	Zeina -	Beautiful, graceful
95.	Ziad -	Abundance
96.	Zoya -	Alive, life
97.	Zuhair -	Bright, shining
98.	Akil -	Intelligent, thoughtful
99.	Amira -	Princess, leader
100.	Nour -	Light

Kuwaiti baby names and their meanings

1. Abdullah - Servant of God
2. Abeer - Fragrance
3. Adel - Just
4. Afra - Dust-colored
5. Ahmed - Much praised
6. Aisha - Living
7. Ali - Elevated
8. Amal - Hope
9. Amani - Wishes
10. Amira - Princess
11. Anwar - Light
12. Asma - Supreme
13. Aziz - Powerful
14. Badr - Full moon
15. Bahija - Joyful
16. Basim - Smiling
17. Batul - Ascetic Virgin
18. Bilal - Water
19. Bushra - Good news
20. Dalia - Vine
21. Dalal - Pampered
22. Fahad - Cheetah
23. Faisal - Decisive
24. Fatima - One who abstains
25. Fawzi - Victorious
26. Fida - Redemption
27. Ghada - Graceful
28. Hadi - Guide
29. Hala - Halo
30. Hamad - Praise
31. Hanan - Compassionate
32. Hassan - Handsome
33. Haya - Life
34. Huda - Guidance

35. Ibrahim - Father of many
36. Iman - Faith
37. Isra - Nocturnal journey
38. Jamal - Beauty
39. Jana - Harvest
40. Jawad - Generous
41. Kamil - Perfect
42. Khalid - Eternal
43. Khadija - Premature child
44. Laila - Night
45. Latif - Gentle
46. Layla - Night
47. Lubna - Storax tree
48. Maha - Wild cow
49. Majed - Glorious
50. Malak - Angel
51. Mariam - Sea of bitterness
52. Mohammed - Praiseworthy
53. Mona - Wishes
54. Nada - Dew
55. Nadia - Caller
56. Nasser - Victorious
57. Nawal - Gift
58. Nawaf - High, lofty
59. Nizar - Little
60. Noor - Light
61. Omar - Long-lived
62. Qasim - Divider
63. Rabab - White cloud
64. Raja - Hope
65. Rashid - Rightly guided
66. Rima - White antelope
67. Rola - Vision
68. Sabah - Morning
69. Saeed - Happy
70. Salim - Safe

71. Sami - Elevated
72. Sara - Princess
73. Shadi - Singer
74. Shaima - Good news
75. Sharif - Noble
76. Suhail - Canopus star
77. Tariq - Morning star
78. Thana - Praise
79. Umar - Life
80. Wafa - Loyalty
81. Walid - Newborn
82. Yasmin - Jasmine
83. Youssef - God will add
84. Zahra - Flowering
85. Zain - Beauty
86. Zainab - Fragrant plant
87. Zaki - Pure
88. Zara - Flower
89. Zein - Graceful
90. Ziad - Increase
91. Hikmat - Wisdom
92. Ibtihaj - Joy
93. Jafar - Stream
94. Kamal - Perfection
95. Lina - Palm tree
96. Muna - Desire
97. Nabil - Noble
98. Rana - Gazing
99. Salwa - Consolation
100. Yara - Small butterfly

Emirati baby names and their meanings

1. Aaban - Name of the Angel
2. Aabid - Worshiper
3. Aahil - Prince
4. Aali - High, noble
5. Aasim - One who restrains
6. Abdul - Servant of God
7. Abdullah - Servant of Allah
8. Abeer - Fragrance
9. Abir - Perfume
10. Adel - Just, upright
11. Adnan - Settler
12. Ahmad - Most commendable
13. Akram - Most generous
14. Ali - Exalted, noble
15. Ameen - Faithful, trustworthy
16. Amjad - More glorious
17. Anas - Affection, love
18. Aqeel - Wise, intelligent
19. Arif - Knowing, aware
20. Asad - Lion
21. Asim - Protector, guardian
22. Ayman - Blessed, lucky
23. Aziz - Powerful, beloved
24. Badr - Full moon
25. Bahir - Dazzling, brilliant
26. Basim - Smiling
27. Bilal - Water, freshness
28. Daanish - Wisdom, learning
29. Dawood - Beloved
30. Ehsan - Perfection, excellence
31. Fahad - Lynx
32. Faisal - Decisive
33. Faris - Horseman, knight
34. Fawaz - Successful

35. Faysal - Resolute
36. Ghazi - Conqueror
37. Hadi - Guide to righteousness
38. Hamad - Praiseworthy
39. Hamdan - Praised
40. Hamid - Praiseworthy
41. Haris - Guardian, protector
42. Hasan - Beautiful, good
43. Hashim - Destroyer of evil
44. Hussain - Handsome, beautiful
45. Ibrahim - Father of multitude
46. Idris - Studious person
47. Imran - Prosperity
48. Irfan - Thankfulness
49. Ismail - God will hear
50. Jamal - Beauty
51. Jawad - Generous
52. Jibril - Archangel Gabriel
53. Kadir - Powerful
54. Kamal - Perfection
55. Karim - Generous
56. Khalid - Eternal
57. Khurram - Delighted
58. Latif - Gentle, kind
59. Madani - Civilized
60. Majid - Noble, glorious
61. Malik - King
62. Mansoor - Victorious
63. Mohsin - Beneficent
64. Mustafa - Chosen one
65. Nabeel - Noble
66. Nadeem - Companion, friend
67. Naseer - Helper
68. Nasser - Victorious
69. Nawaf - High, lofty
70. Omar - Long-lived

71. Qasim - One who distributes
72. Rafiq - Kind, friend
73. Rashid - Rightly-guided
74. Raza - Contentment
75. Rehan - Scented
76. Saad - Good luck
77. Sabir - Patient
78. Sadiq - Truthful
79. Safwan - Rock
80. Salah - Righteousness
81. Salim - Safe, sound
82. Salman - Safe
83. Sami - Exalted, sublime
84. Saeed - Happy, fortunate
85. Taha - A name of the Prophet Muhammad
86. Taimur - Iron
87. Talib - Seeker
88. Tariq - Morning star
89. Umar - Life, long living
90. Usman - The young of a bird
91. Wael - Seeker of refuge
92. Waleed - Newborn child
93. Yasin - A chapter of the Quran
94. Yasir - Wealthy
95. Youssef - God will add
96. Yaqub - Supplanter
97. Zafar - Victory
98. Zaid - To prosper
99. Zain - Beauty, grace
100. Ziyad - Growth, progress

Qatari baby names and their meanings

1. Aaliyah - High, exalted
2. Abdullah - Servant of God
3. Abir - Fragrance
4. Adel - Just, fair
5. Ahlam - Dreams
6. Ahmed - Highly praised
7. Aisha - Living, prosperous
8. Akram - Most generous
9. Alia - Exalted, noble
10. Amal - Hope, expectation
11. Ammar - Long-living
12. Amna - Peaceful, safe
13. Anas - Affection, love
14. Aseel - Noble, highborn
15. Asma - Supreme, exalted
16. Ayman - Lucky, right-handed
17. Badr - Full moon
18. Basma - A smile
19. Bilal - Water, moisture
20. Bushra - Good news
21. Dalia - Branch, vine
22. Dana - Pearl
23. Farah - Joy, happiness
24. Farid - Unique, singular
25. Fatima - Daughter of the Prophet
26. Fawaz - Successful
27. Faisal - Decisive
28. Ghada - Graceful woman
29. Habib - Beloved
30. Hadi - Guide to righteousness
31. Hala - Halo around the moon
32. Hamad - Praiseworthy
33. Hanan - Mercy, compassion
34. Hassan - Handsome, good

35. Haya - Life
36. Ibrahim - Father of many
37. Iman - Faith, belief
38. Irfan - Gratefulness
39. Isra - Night journey
40. Jamal - Beauty
41. Jana - Harvest
42. Jawad - Generous
43. Kader - Powerful
44. Khalid - Eternal, immortal
45. Khadija - Early baby
46. Laila - Night
47. Latifa - Gentle, kind
48. Layla - Night, born at night
49. Leena - Tender
50. Lubna - Storax tree
51. Mahdi - Guided one
52. Mahmud - Praised
53. Maha - Wild cow, deer
54. Malik - King, owner
55. Mariam - Lady, mistress
56. Marwan - Solid
57. Mona - Wishes, desires
58. Musa - Saved from the water
59. Nada - Generosity, dew
60. Nadia - Caller
61. Nafisa - Precious gem
62. Nahla - Drink of water
63. Nasser - Helper, supporter
64. Noor - Light
65. Omar - Life, long-lived
66. Qasim - Divider, distributor
67. Rabia - Spring
68. Radwan - Pleasure, satisfaction
69. Rana - Gazing, looking at
70. Rasha - Young gazelle

71. Rashid - Rightly guided
72. Reem - Gazelle
73. Riad - Gardens, meadows
74. Rida - Contentment, satisfaction
75. Rima - White antelope
76. Saba - Morning
77. Sabah - Morning
78. Sabir - Patient
79. Saif - Sword
80. Salma - Peaceful, safe
81. Sami - Elevated, sublime
82. Sara - Noble lady
83. Tariq - Morning star
84. Umar - Life, long-lived
85. Wafa - Loyalty
86. Yahya - God is gracious
87. Yasmin - Jasmine flower
88. Youssef - God will increase
89. Zahra - Flower, beauty
90. Zaid - Growth, abundance
91. Zaina - Beauty, grace
92. Zara - Blooming flower
93. Zayed - Growth, abundance
94. Zeinab - Fragrant flower
95. Ziya - Light, glow
96. Zuhair - Bright, shining
97. Zain - Beauty, grace
98. Zaki - Pure
99. Ziad - Abundance, growth
100. Zulaikha - Brilliant beauty

Omani baby names and their meanings

1. Abdullah - Servant of God
2. Ahmed - Highly praised
3. Aisha - Living, prosperous
4. Ali - Exalted, noble
5. Amira - Princess
6. Ayaan - Gift of God
7. Badr - Full moon
8. Barakah - Blessing
9. Bilal - Water, freshness
10. Dalia - Flower
11. Emir - Prince, ruler
12. Fahad - Leopard
13. Fatima - Daughter of Prophet Muhammad
14. Ghazi - Warrior
15. Habiba - Beloved
16. Hamza - Lion
17. Hasan - Good, handsome
18. Huda - Right guidance
19. Ibrahim - Father of many
20. Iman - Faith
21. Jamal - Beauty
22. Jannah - Paradise
23. Kareem - Generous
24. Khalid - Eternal
25. Layla - Night
26. Malik - King
27. Mariam - Sea of bitterness
28. Nasser - Victory
29. Noor - Light
30. Omar - Life
31. Qasim - Divider
32. Rabia - Spring
33. Safiya - Pure
34. Tariq - Morning star

35. Umar - Long-lived
36. Yasmin - Jasmine
37. Zainab - Fragrant flower
38. Zaki - Pure
39. Abeer - Fragrance
40. Adnan - Settler
41. Afra - Color of earth
42. Amin - Trustworthy
43. Basma - Smile
44. Dalal - Touched in a kind and loving way
45. Ehsan - Charity
46. Fadil - Generous
47. Ghada - Graceful
48. Hafsa - Lioness
49. Ibtisam - Smile
50. Jafar - Stream
51. Kamil - Perfect
52. Latifa - Gentle, kind
53. Muna - Wish, desire
54. Naima - Comfort, tranquility
55. Qamar - Moon
56. Rashid - Righteous
57. Salim - Safe
58. Taha - A name of Prophet Muhammad
59. Uthman - Baby bustard
60. Yara - Small butterfly
61. Zahra - Flower
62. Ziyad - Growth
63. Adel - Just
64. Bahija - Joyful
65. Daud - Beloved
66. Faisal - Decisive
67. Hani - Happy
68. Idris - Studious
69. Jalal - Majesty
70. Kader - Powerful

71. Lina - Tender
72. Majid - Noble
73. Nabil - Noble
74. Osama - Lion
75. Rania - Gazing
76. Sami - High, elevated
77. Taimur - Iron
78. Wafa - Faithfulness
79. Yasin - The two opening letters of Surah 36 in the Quran
80. Zahid - Ascetic
81. Asma - Supreme
82. Bilqis - Queen of Sheba
83. Dina - Judged
84. Farid - Unique
85. Huda - Right guidance
86. Iqbal - Prosperity
87. Jamal - Beauty
88. Kamal - Perfection
89. Lulu - Pearl
90. Mansoor - Victorious
91. Nadia - Caller
92. Othman - Companion of the Prophet
93. Rahim - Merciful
94. Salma - Peaceful
95. Tariq - Morning star
96. Waleed - Newborn child
97. Yasir - Wealthy
98. Zara - Blooming flower
99. Asif - Gather
100. Barir - Faithful

Bahraini baby names and their meanings

1. Aali - Exalted, high and superior
2. Abdul - Servant of God
3. Adnan - Settled or permanent
4. Ahmed - Highly praised or one who praises
5. Ali - Noble, sublime, and exalted
6. Amal - Hope or expectation
7. Amina - Trustworthy, faithful
8. Amira - Princess, leader
9. Arif - Knowledgeable, wise
10. Asma - Supreme or exalted
11. Aziz - Powerful, respected
12. Bahar - Spring or bloom
13. Basim - Smiling, cheerful
14. Batul - Ascetic virgin
15. Bilal - Water, freshness
16. Bushra - Good news
17. Dalia - Branch or vine
18. Daud - Beloved, dear
19. Eman - Faith, belief
20. Fadil - Generous, honorable
21. Faisal - Decisive, judge
22. Fatima - Daughter of the Prophet, captivating
23. Fawzi - Victorious, successful
24. Ghada - Graceful, young woman
25. Habib - Beloved, dear
26. Hadi - Guide to righteousness
27. Hafsa - Lion's cub, young lion
28. Hala - Halo around the moon
29. Hamad - Praised, commendable
30. Hanan - Mercy, compassion
31. Hasan - Handsome, good
32. Hawa - Love, affection
33. Ibrahim - Father of many
34. Idris - Studious, knowledgeable

35. Iman - Faith, belief
36. Jamal - Beauty, grace
37. Jawad - Generous, liberal
38. Kamil - Perfect, complete
39. Karim - Generous, noble
40. Khalid - Eternal, immortal
41. Khadija - Premature child
42. Laila - Night, dark beauty
43. Latif - Gentle, kind
44. Layla - Night, dark beauty
45. Lubna - Storax tree
46. Maha - Wild cow, deer
47. Mahdi - Guided to the right path
48. Majid - Noble, glorious
49. Malik - King, ruler
50. Mariam - Sea of bitterness
51. Marwa - Fragrant plant
52. Maryam - Bitter, sea of bitterness
53. Muna - Wish, desire
54. Nadia - Caller, announcer
55. Naim - Comfort, tranquility
56. Najwa - Secret conversation
57. Nawal - Gift, present
58. Nizar - Little
59. Noor - Light, radiance
60. Omar - Life, long living
61. Qasim - Divider, distributor
62. Rabia - Spring, fourth
63. Rahim - Merciful, compassionate
64. Rashid - Rightly guided
65. Rida - Contentment, satisfaction
66. Rima - White antelope
67. Sabah - Morning
68. Sabir - Patient, enduring
69. Salim - Safe, sound
70. Samir - Entertaining companion

71. Sana - Brilliance, radiance
72. Sara - Princess
73. Sharif - Noble, honored
74. Suhail - Gentle, easy
75. Taha - A name of the Prophet Muhammad
76. Talal - Admirable, nice
77. Tamim - Complete, perfect
78. Tariq - Morning star
79. Umar - Flourishing, thriving
80. Wafa - Loyalty, faithfulness
81. Yahya - God is gracious
82. Yasir - Wealthy, prosperous
83. Yusuf - God will add
84. Zain - Grace, beauty
85. Zainab - Fragrant flower
86. Zaki - Pure, chaste
87. Zara - Blooming flower
88. Zein - Good, beautiful
89. Abdullah - Servant of God
90. Aisha - Alive, she who lives
91. Ayman - Lucky, right-handed
92. Haya - Life, existence
93. Jamal - Beauty
94. Jannah - Paradise, heaven
95. Khaled - Immortal, eternal
96. Layla - Night, dark beauty
97. Malak - Angel
98. Nada - Generosity, dew
99. Noora - Light, illumination
100. Zayed - Grower, increaser

Pakistani baby names and their meanings

1. Aaban - Name of the angel
2. Aabid - Worshipper
3. Aabir - Fragrance
4. Aabish - Daughter of Sa'd who was a queen of Iran
5. Aabroo - Honor, dignity
6. Aadam - The first prophet of Allah
7. Aadeel - Just
8. Aadil - Just, Upright
9. Aadila - Just, Honest, Equal
10. Aafa - Forgiver
11. Aafreen - Brave, Acclaim
12. Aahil - Prince
13. Aaida - Visiting, Returning
14. Aaima - Leader, Ruler
15. Aaira - Noble, Respectful
16. Aaisha - Life, Vivaciousness
17. Aalam - World, Universe
18. Aalee - Sublime, High
19. Aaleyah - Exalted, Highest social standing
20. Aalim - Scholar, Authority
21. Aalina - Beautiful, noble
22. Aaliyah - Tall, Towering
23. Aamaal - Hopes, Aspirations
24. Aamanee - Good wish
25. Aamil - Doer, Work man
26. Aamina - Mother of Prophet Muhammad
27. Aamir - Civilised
28. Aamirah - Inhabitant
29. Aaqib - Follower
30. Aaqil - Intelligent
31. Aara - Adoring
32. Aarib - Handsome, healthy
33. Aarif - Knowing, Aware
34. Aarifa - Learned, Expert

35. Aariz - Respectable man
36. Aarzoo - Wish
37. Aas - Hope
38. Aasi - Hopeful
39. Aasim - Person who restrains
40. Aasiyah - The Muslim wife of Pharaoh
41. Aasma - Excellent, Precious
42. Aatif - Kind, Affectionate
43. Aatifa - Affectionate, Compassionate
44. Aatik - Pure, Clean
45. Aatika - Lady who is richly perfumed
46. Aatir - Fragrant
47. Aatifah - Compassionate, Affectionate
48. Aaus - Name of a tree
49. Aayan - Gift of God
50. Aayat - Verses in the Quran
51. Aayun - Springs, Wells
52. Abaan - Old Arabic name
53. Abad - Father
54. Abadiya - Ibn al Abadiyah was an author
55. Aban - Old Arabic name
56. Abasi - Stern
57. Abbas - Lion
58. Abbiah - God is my father
59. Abbu - Father
60. Abdah - Worshipper of Allah
61. Abdal - Servant of Allah
62. Abdallah - Servant of God
63. Abdeali - Follower of Ali
64. Abdel - Servant
65. Abdellatif - Servant of the gentle
66. Abdhut - Unique
67. Abdi - My servant
68. Abdia - Gift of God
69. Abdil - Servant
70. Abdish - Noble, Unique

71. Abdu - Servant of God
72. Abdullah - Servant of Allah
73. Abeed - Worshipper of Allah
74. Abeel - Healthy
75. Abeera - The mixture of the smell of the petals of rose and sundal
76. Abeesha - Gift of God
77. Abha - Brightness
78. Abhaya - Fearless
79. Abia - Great
80. Abid - Worshipper of God
81. Abida - Worshipper
82. Abidah - Worshipper
83. Abidah - Worshipper of Allah
84. Abidur - Worshipper
85. Abir - Fragrance
86. Abira - Strong
87. Abirah - Fleeting, transitory, ephemeral
88. Abisana - Brilliant, Magnificent, Shining
89. Abla - Perfectly formed
90. Abood - Worshipper of Allah
91. Abqurah - Genius
92. Abrad - Cold, Clouds
93. Abrar - Devoted to God
94. Abraha - From Abir, fragrance
95. Abrash - Spotted, Speckled
96. Absar - Vision, Sight
97. Absat - Wide, vast, spacious
98. Abtahi - Born in Ghazva
99. Abul - Father
100. Abul Khayr - One who does good

Bangladeshi baby names and their meanings

1. Aahna - Exist
2. Aarav - Peaceful
3. Abir - Fragrance
4. Aditi - Free and unbounded
5. Afsana - Story
6. Ahaan - Dawn
7. Alisha - Protected by God
8. Aliza - Joyful
9. Anaya - Caring
10. Anik - Soldier
11. Anika - Grace
12. Anis - Close friend
13. Anika - Graceful
14. Anis - Companion
15. Arham - Merciful
16. Arisha - Highness
17. Arnav - Ocean
18. Asha - Hope
19. Ashiq - Lover
20. Asif - Gather
21. Asma - Supreme
22. Ayaan - Gift of God
23. Ayat - Verse
24. Ayman - Lucky
25. Azad - Free
26. Azim - Great
27. Baha - Beautiful
28. Bari - Creator
29. Barir - Faithful
30. Basma - Smile
31. Bina - Understanding
32. Bushra - Good news
33. Dia - Light

34. Ehsan - Charitable
35. Elma - Apple
36. Fahad - Lynx
37. Farah - Joy
38. Fariha - Happy
39. Faris - Horseman
40. Fatima - Daughter of the Prophet
41. Faysal - Judge
42. Gazal - Song
43. Habib - Beloved
44. Hafsa - Cub
45. Hani - Happy
46. Hasan - Handsome
47. Hasna - Beautiful
48. Haya - Modesty
49. Iman - Faith
50. Inaya - Caring
51. Iqra - Read
52. Isra - Night journey
53. Jannat - Heaven
54. Javed - Eternal
55. Kainat - Universe
56. Kamal - Perfection
57. Karim - Generous
58. Khaled - Eternal
59. Lina - Tender
60. Mahi - Fish
61. Mahir - Skilled
62. Maisha - Life
63. Majed - Glorious
64. Malika - Queen
65. Manha - Gift of Allah
66. Maruf - Known
67. Maryam - Name of Prophet's Daughter
68. Masud - Happy
69. Mina - Love

70. Mirza - Prince
71. Misbah - Lamp
72. Misha - Smile
73. Nabil - Noble
74. Nadia - Caller
75. Nafisa - Precious
76. Nahid - Generous
77. Naim - Comfort
78. Naira - Shining
79. Najma - Star
80. Naveed - Good news
81. Nazia - Pride
82. Nida - Call
83. Nihad - Height
84. Nila - Sapphire
85. Noor - Light
86. Omar - Life
87. Parvez - Success
88. Qamar - Moon
89. Rahim - Compassionate
90. Rahman - Merciful
91. Raihan - Fragrance
92. Raisa - Leader
93. Rana - Gazing
94. Rania - Queen
95. Rashid - Guided
96. Rida - Contentment
97. Sabrina - Princess
98. Safa - Purity
99. Sami - Exalted
100. Zara - Princess

Sri Lankan baby names and their meanings

1. Aadhya - First power
2. Aarav - Peaceful
3. Abhinav - Brand new
4. Adhira - Lightning
5. Advaith - Unique
6. Ahana - Dawn
7. Aishwarya - Wealth
8. Akila - Intelligent
9. Amara - Eternal
10. Amrita - Immortality
11. Anaya - Caring
12. Anika - Grace
13. Ansh - Portion
14. Anuja - Younger sister
15. Arnav - Ocean
16. Arya - Noble
17. Asha - Hope
18. Ashoka - Without sorrow
19. Atul - Incomparable
20. Avani - Earth
21. Avantika - Queen
22. Ayush - Long-lived
23. Bhavana - Feelings
24. Bhavya - Grand
25. Chaitanya - Consciousness
26. Chandana - Sandalwood
27. Charu - Beautiful
28. Daksha - Able
29. Darshana - Vision
30. Deepa - Light
31. Devi - Goddess
32. Dhanya - Thankful
33. Dheer - Patient
34. Ekta - Unity

35. Esha - Desire
36. Gauri - White
37. Girish - Lord of mountains
38. Harsha - Happiness
39. Hema - Golden
40. Indra - King of gods
41. Ishani - Desire
42. Jagath - Universe
43. Janani - Mother
44. Jayani - Conqueror
45. Kalyani - Auspicious
46. Kanishka - Small
47. Karishma - Miracle
48. Kavindu - Moon of poets
49. Keshini - One with beautiful hair
50. Lakshmi - Goddess of wealth
51. Lathika - Small creeper
52. Madhavi - Sweet
53. Mahesh - Great ruler
54. Malini - Fragrant
55. Manjula - Lovely
56. Nalini - Lotus
57. Nandini - Daughter
58. Naveen - New
59. Nihara - Mist
60. Nishad - Seventh note on Indian musical scale
61. Ojas - Strength
62. Padma - Lotus
63. Prabha - Light
64. Pradeep - Light
65. Pranav - Sacred syllable Om
66. Priya - Loved one
67. Radha - Successful
68. Ravi - Sun
69. Roshan - Bright
70. Saachi - Truth

71. Sachin - Pure
72. Saman - Equal
73. Sandhya - Twilight
74. Sanjana - Gentle
75. Saraswati - Goddess of knowledge
76. Sathya - Truth
77. Shanti - Peace
78. Shreya - Beautiful
79. Sita - Furrow
80. Subha - Auspicious
81. Sudha - Nectar
82. Suman - Flower
83. Sumitra - Good friend
84. Suraj - Sun
85. Surya - Sun
86. Swati - Star
87. Tanvi - Slender
88. Tejas - Brightness
89. Uday - To rise
90. Usha - Dawn
91. Vaibhav - Prosperity
92. Varun - God of water
93. Veena - A musical instrument
94. Vidya - Knowledge
95. Vijay - Victory
96. Vinay - Modesty
97. Vishnu - Preserver of universe
98. Yash - Fame
99. Yeshi - Brave
100. Zara - Princess

Nepali baby names and their meanings

1. Aarav - Peaceful
2. Abhinav - New, young, fresh
3. Aditya - Sun
4. Alisha - Protected by God
5. Anika - Grace
6. Anish - Supreme
7. Anjali - Offering with both hands
8. Anuradha - A bright star
9. Arjun - Bright, shining, white
10. Asha - Hope
11. Avinash - Indestructible
12. Ayesha - Alive, well-living
13. Bimal - Pure
14. Bina - Understanding, wisdom
15. Bishnu - The preserver
16. Chandra - Moon
17. Deepa - Light, lamp
18. Dinesh - Sun
19. Ekta - Unity
20. Gita - Song
21. Gyan - Knowledge
22. Harish - Lord Vishnu
23. Indira - Beauty
24. Ishan - Sun
25. Jaya - Victory
26. Kabita - Poem
27. Kailash - Name of a Himalayan peak, abode of Lord Shiva
28. Kamal - Lotus
29. Keshav - Another name of Lord Krishna
30. Krishna - Dark, black
31. Laxmi - Goddess of wealth
32. Madan - God of love
33. Madhav - Sweet like honey

34. Manish - God of the mind
35. Maya - Illusion
36. Mohan - Charming, fascinating
37. Nabin - New
38. Nandini - Daughter
39. Narendra - King of men
40. Nisha - Night
41. Om - Sacred syllable in Hinduism
42. Pooja - Worship
43. Prakash - Light
44. Pramod - Happiness
45. Priya - Beloved
46. Raj - Rule, kingdom
47. Rama - Pleasing
48. Ramesh - Lord Rama
49. Rani - Queen
50. Rita - Truthful
51. Rohit - Red
52. Sagar - Ocean
53. Sajjan - Good man
54. Samir - Wind
55. Sandhya - Evening
56. Sanjay - Victorious
57. Sarita - River
58. Shanti - Peace
59. Shiva - The auspicious one
60. Shyam - Dark, black
61. Sita - Furrow
62. Suman - Flower
63. Suraj - Sun
64. Suresh - Ruler of the gods
65. Sweta - Fair
66. Tara - Star
67. Uday - To rise
68. Usha - Dawn
69. Vijay - Victory

70. Vinod - Happy
71. Yamuna - Jamuna River
72. Yash - Glory, fame
73. Abir - Strong
74. Aditi - Freedom, security
75. Akash - Sky
76. Amrita - Immortality
77. Anil - Air, wind
78. Anuja - Younger sister
79. Apsara - Celestial maiden
80. Arati - Hymns sung in praise of god
81. Bhanu - Sun
82. Bhaskar - Sun
83. Bijay - Victorious
84. Chetana - Consciousness
85. Dev - God
86. Durga - Unreachable
87. Esha - Desire
88. Gauri - Fair
89. Hema - Golden
90. Indu - Moon
91. Jeevan - Life
92. Kanti - Light
93. Lalita - Beautiful woman
94. Mala - Garland
95. Nanda - Joy
96. Padma - Lotus
97. Radha - Successful
98. Rupa - Silver
99. Sunita - Well-behaved
100. Trishna - Thirst

Bhutanese baby names and their meanings

1. Choki -   peaceful
2. Tenzin -   upholder of teachings
3. Pema -   lotus
4. Sonam -   fortunate or lucky
5. Dorji -   thunderbolt
6. Tashi -   auspicious
7. Jigme -   fearless
8. Wangchuk -   power of the thunderbolt
9. Norbu -   jewel
10. Lhaden -   fortunate and prosperous
11. Kuenzang -   universal goodness
12. Kinley -   kind heart
13. Dechen -   great bliss
14. Yeshey -   wisdom
15. Ugyen -   representative of the Buddha
16. Rinchen -   precious gem
17. Sangay -   Buddha
18. Phuntsho -   abundance
19. Zangmo -   good woman
20. Tshering -   longevity
21. Karma -   action or deed
22. Choden -   devout
23. Lhagyal -   successful
24. Tandin -   upholder of the teachings
25. Tsedrup -   religious practice
26. Gyeltshen -   victorious banner
27. Zam -   path
28. Chime -   immortal
29. Rigden -   holder of knowledge
30. Dawa -   moon
31. Phub -   to grow
32. Lhamo -   goddess
33. Yonten -   knowledgeable
34. Tobgay -   successful and meritorious

35. Kelsang - good times
36. Drakpa - brave
37. Yangchen - melodious voice
38. Pelden - glorious
39. Namgyel - victorious in all directions
40. Thinley - ethical behavior
41. Tsagay - eloquent speaker
42. Zangpo - good man
43. Gyem - jewel
44. Phurba - ritual dagger
45. Lhundup - spontaneous
46. Jamtsho - friend of the world
47. Dorjee - indestructible
48. Tshomo - female
49. Samdrup - fulfilling wishes
50. Tshewang - power
51. Tshultrim - righteous
52. Kesang - good fortune
53. Chundu - god of the universe
54. Wangmo - queen
55. Jampa - loving kindness
56. Tsheten - stable
57. Damchoe - supreme dharma
58. Gyembo - king
59. Tshoki - religious
60. Singye - lion
61. Loday - intelligent
62. Chimi - immortal
63. Yeshi - wisdom
64. Zeko - victorious
65. Samten - meditation
66. Tshering - long life
67. Lhawang - power
68. Chophel - dharma flourishing
69. Tshewang - power
70. Tandin - upholder of the teachings

71. Pem - lotus
72. Tshokey - light of dharma
73. Tobden - truth
74. Wangdi - power
75. Gyem - jewel
76. Tsheyang - long life and prosperity
77. Zangley - good heart
78. Dendup - increase
79. Sonam - merit
80. Tashi - auspicious
81. Thrinley - karma
82. Dorji - diamond
83. Choki - peaceful
84. Jigme - fearless
85. Wangchuk - king
86. Norbu - jewel
87. Lhaden - fortunate and prosperous
88. Kuenzang - universal goodness
89. Kinley - kind heart
90. Dechen - great bliss
91. Yeshey - wisdom
92. Ugyen - representative of the Buddha
93. Rinchen - precious gem
94. Sangay - Buddha
95. Phuntsho - abundance
96. Zangmo - good woman
97. Tshering - longevity
98. Karma - action or deed
99. Choden - devout
100. Lhagyal - successful

Afghan baby names and their meanings

1. Abdullah - Servant of God
2. Aisha - Alive
3. Ali - Exalted
4. Amina - Trustworthy
5. Asad - Lion
6. Ayub - Patient
7. Aziz - Powerful
8. Bahar - Spring
9. Baran - Rain
10. Basir - Insightful
11. Bilal - Water
12. Daud - Beloved
13. Delara - Adorning the heart
14. Elham - Inspiration
15. Farah - Joy
16. Farid - Unique
17. Fatima - Daughter of the Prophet
18. Feroz - Successful
19. Gul - Flower
20. Habib - Beloved
21. Hafsa - Lioness
22. Hakim - Wise
23. Hamid - Praiseworthy
24. Hana - Happiness
25. Haroon - High or exalted
26. Hasina - Beautiful
27. Hayat - Life
28. Husna - Beauty
29. Idris - Studious
30. Imran - Prosperity
31. Iqbal - Prosperity
32. Jamal - Beauty
33. Jamila - Beautiful
34. Javed - Eternal

35. Kamil - Perfect
36. Karim - Generous
37. Khadija - Premature child
38. Khalid - Eternal
39. Layla - Night
40. Lina - Tender
41. Mahdi - Guided one
42. Mahir - Skilled
43. Mina - Love
44. Mirwais - Light of the home
45. Mohammed - Praised one
46. Mujtaba - Chosen one
47. Nadia - Caller
48. Najib - Noble
49. Nasim - Breeze
50. Nasrin - Wild rose
51. Omar - Long-lived
52. Parisa - Like a fairy
53. Qasim - Divider
54. Rahim - Merciful
55. Rahman - Compassionate
56. Rashid - Rightly guided
57. Raza - Contentment
58. Reza - Contentment
59. Roshan - Bright
60. Saad - Good luck
61. Sabir - Patient
62. Sadaf - Pearl
63. Saeed - Happy
64. Safa - Pure
65. Sami - Elevated
66. Samira - Entertaining companion
67. Sara - Pure
68. Shabnam - Dew
69. Shahid - Witness
70. Shakila - Beautiful

71. Shams - Sun
72. Sharif - Noble
73. Shireen - Sweet
74. Sohail - Star
75. Soraya - Princess
76. Tariq - Morning star
77. Tasneem - A spring in paradise
78. Umar - Flourishing
79. Wahid - Unique
80. Yasmin - Jasmine flower
81. Yousuf - God will increase
82. Zahra - Flower
83. Zainab - Father's jewel
84. Zahir - Bright, shining
85. Zaki - Pure
86. Zaman - Time, age
87. Zara - Flower
88. Zia - Light
89. Zohra - Venus
90. Zubair - Strong, powerful
91. Aman - Security, peace
92. Ayan - Gift of God
93. Bano - Lady, princess
94. Darya - Sea
95. Ehsan - Charitable
96. Farzan - Wise
97. Gulzar - Rose garden
98. Iman - Faith
99. Jawad - Generous
100. Laila - Night beauty

Kazakhstani baby names and their meanings

1. Aigul - Moon flower
2. Aisulu - Beautiful moon
3. Akbota - White swan
4. Akmaral - White deer
5. Alima - Wise
6. Altyn - Gold
7. Altynay - Golden moon
8. Amina - Trustworthy
9. Anara - Pomegranate
10. Aruzhan - Beautiful soul
11. Asel - Honey
12. Asima - Protector
13. Asiya - Healer
14. Ayana - Beautiful flower
15. Aygul - Moon rose
16. Ayim - Moon
17. Bagdat - Gift of God
18. Bakhyt - Happiness
19. Balnur - Radiant honey
20. Bibigul - Lady rose
21. Bolat - Steel
22. Botagoz - Pearl eye
23. Damir - Give peace
24. Danel - God is my judge
25. Dariga - Wealthy
26. Dinara - Gold coin
27. Duman - Mist
28. Edil - Noble
29. Erke - Girl
30. Erzhan - Soul of a leader
31. Farida - Unique
32. Galym - Great
33. Gulmira - Miracle rose
34. Gulnara - Pomegranate flower

35. Gulnaz - Proud like a rose
36. Gulzhan - Flower soul
37. Ilyas - The Lord is my God
38. Indira - Beauty
39. Inkar - Refusal
40. Islam - Submission to God
41. Jazira - Island
42. Kamila - Perfect
43. Kanat - Wing
44. Kassym - Share
45. Kymbat - Dream
46. Madina - City of the Prophet
47. Makpal - Protected
48. Malika - Queen
49. Marzhan - Coral
50. Merey - Prosperity
51. Mira - Peace
52. Moldir - Creator
53. Nargul - Pomegranate flower
54. Nazerke - Seeing beauty
55. Nurai - Radiant
56. Nuray - Radiant moon
57. Nurzhan - Radiant soul
58. Perizat - Fairy
59. Raushan - Light
60. Sabina - Beautiful
61. Saule - Sun
62. Serik - Supporter
63. Sholpan - Morning star
64. Sultan - Ruler
65. Tair - Bird
66. Tamara - Palm tree
67. Tolegen - Son of iron
68. Tomiris - Queen
69. Ulzhan - Radiant soul
70. Umut - Hope

71. Yerbolat - Strong like steel
72. Yerkali - Strong man
73. Zere - Gold
74. Zhanar - Pomegranate flower
75. Zhanat - Paradise
76. Zhansaya - Soul of the people
77. Zhasmina - Jasmine
78. Zhibek - Silk
79. Zhuldyz - Star
80. Aidos - Modesty
81. Aigerim - Moonlight
82. Aidana - Moon
83. Aigul - Moonflower
84. Ainur - Moonlight
85. Akniet - Snowdrop
86. Akzhol - White path
87. Aliya - Exalted
88. Almas - Diamond
89. Altynshash - Golden beauty
90. Amina - Safe
91. Aray - Beautiful soul
92. Aruzhan - Beautiful soul
93. Asan - Easy
94. Asel - Honey
95. Askhat - Name of a star
96. Asiya - Consolation
97. Ayazhan - Moon soul
98. Aydana - Moon
99. Aynur - Moonlight
100. Azhar - Flowers

Uzbekistani baby names and their meanings

1. Adolat - Fairness
2. Alisher - Lion of God
3. Amira - Princess
4. Anora - Pomegranate
5. Aziza - Precious
6. Bahodir - Brave
7. Bakhtiyor - Fortunate
8. Botir - Hero
9. Dildora - Heart's pearl
10. Dilfuza - Heart's delight
11. Dilshod - Happy heart
12. Elbek - Powerful
13. Elmira - Princess
14. Erkin - Free
15. Fazliddin - Grace of faith
16. Feruza - Turquoise
17. Gulnora - Pomegranate flower
18. Gulshan - Rose garden
19. Gulzar - Flower garden
20. Habiba - Beloved
21. Hamida - Praiseworthy
22. Hasina - Beautiful
23. Ibrohim - Father of many
24. Iftikhar - Honor
25. Ilhom - Inspiration
26. Ismoil - God will hear
27. Jasur - Brave
28. Kamila - Perfect
29. Karim - Generous
30. Khurshid - Sun
31. Komila - Complete
32. Latif - Gentle
33. Laylo - Night
34. Madina - City of the Prophet

35. Mahbuba - Beloved
36. Mahzuna - Moon
37. Malika - Queen
38. Mansur - Victorious
39. Marhabo - Welcome
40. Mavluda - Born
41. Mekhriniso - Sun's ray
42. Mirzabek - Prince
43. Mukhammad - Praised
44. Munira - Luminous
45. Nargiza - Narcissus flower
46. Nasiba - Noble
47. Nodira - Rare
48. Nafisa - Precious
49. Odil - Justice
50. Oydin - Clear
51. Ozoda - Independent
52. Parvina - Pleiades star cluster
53. Rahima - Merciful
54. Rashid - Rightly guided
55. Ravshan - Bright
56. Sabina - Beautiful
57. Sahiba - Lady
58. Salima - Safe
59. Sanjar - Prince
60. Sarvinoz - Cypress beauty
61. Shakhzoda - Princess
62. Shavkat - Dignity
63. Shirin - Sweet
64. Shohruh - Famous
65. Shukrona - Thankful
66. Sitora - Star
67. Tahir - Pure
68. Tahmina - Strong
69. Tamara - Palm tree
70. Tohir - Pure

71. Umid - Hope
72. Ummid - Hope
73. Vohid - Unique
74. Xurshid - Sun
75. Yulduz - Star
76. Zafar - Victory
77. Zarrin - Golden
78. Zebiniso - Beautiful woman
79. Ziyoda - Independent
80. Zuhra - Venus
81. Zulaykho - Beautiful
82. Zulfizar - Beautiful
83. Abdurahim - Servant of the merciful
84. Adham - Black
85. Akmal - Perfect
86. Alibek - Noble leader
87. Anvar - Brighter
88. Asadbek - Lion prince
89. Azim - Great
90. Bahrom - Spring
91. Bekzod - Prince
92. Daler - Brave
93. Davron - Time
94. Dilshod - Happy heart
95. Elyor - People's friend
96. Farhod - Happiness
97. Firdavs - Paradise
98. Jahongir - World conqueror
99. Jamshid - Sun's shine
100. Zafar - Victory

Tajikistani baby names and their meanings

1. Abdukadir - Servant of the Capable
2. Abduqodir - Servant of the Powerful
3. Akmal - Most complete
4. Alim - Learned, wise
5. Anvar - Bright, luminous
6. Azim - Determined, resolved
7. Bahodur - Brave, courageous
8. Bakhtiyor - Lucky, fortunate
9. Botir - Hero, brave
10. Davron - Time, age
11. Dilshod - Happy heart
12. Elyor - High, lofty
13. Farhod - Happy, joyous
14. Firdavs - Paradise
15. Gulom - Slave, servant
16. Habib - Beloved, darling
17. Ibrohim - Father of many
18. Ismoil - God will hear
19. Jahongir - Conqueror of the world
20. Kamol - Perfection, completeness
21. Khasan - Handsome, good
22. Latif - Gentle, kind
23. Mansur - Victorious, assisted
24. Mirzo - Prince, nobleman
25. Nodir - Rare, precious
26. Otabek - Prince servant
27. Parviz - Happy, lucky
28. Qahramon - Hero, champion
29. Rahim - Merciful, compassionate
30. Rustam - Strong, brave
31. Shavkat - Dignity, power
32. Tohir - Pure, virtuous
33. Umar - Long-lived, flourishing
34. Vahid - Unique, singular

35. Yodgor - Memorable, unforgettable
36. Zafar - Victory, triumph
37. Zohir - Bright, shining
38. Amina - Trustworthy, faithful
39. Aziza - Precious, cherished
40. Bahor - Spring
41. Dilbar - Sweetheart, beloved
42. Farangis - Charming, enchanting
43. Gulnora - Pomegranate light
44. Habiba - Beloved, darling
45. Iftikhar - Pride, glory
46. Jamila - Beautiful, pretty
47. Khurshid - Sun, radiant
48. Lutfiya - Gentle, kind
49. Malika - Queen, sovereign
50. Nargis - Narcissus flower
51. Oisha - Alive, living
52. Parvina - Pleiades star cluster
53. Qizg'on - Love, affection
54. Rahima - Merciful, compassionate
55. Saodat - Happiness, bliss
56. Tahmina - Strong, brave
57. Umid - Hope, expectation
58. Vahida - Unique, singular
59. Yodgora - Memorable, unforgettable
60. Zafira - Victorious, successful
61. Zuhra - Venus, beauty
62. Asal - Honey, sweetness
63. Bahri - Of the sea
64. Dilnoza - Heart's desire
65. Farida - Unique, singular
66. Gulbahor - Spring rose
67. Halima - Gentle, kind
68. Isfandiyar - Pure, clean
69. Javohir - Gem, jewel
70. Khalima - Dream, vision

71. Laylo - Night
72. Munisa - Friendly, sociable
73. Nodira - Rare, precious
74. Oydin - Bright, luminous
75. Parizoda - Fairy child
76. Qumri - Moonlight
77. Rano - Morning
78. Saodat - Happiness, bliss
79. Tahira - Pure, clean
80. Umida - Hope, expectation
81. Vahdat - Unity, oneness
82. Yodgorlik - Memory, remembrance
83. Zarina - Golden
84. Asror - Secrets
85. Botirali - Heroic
86. Davlat - State, country
87. Elnur - Light of the eyes
88. Firdavs - Paradise
89. Gulomjon - Flower servant
90. Habibulloh - Beloved of God
91. Islom - Submission to God
92. Javon - Youth
93. Kholiq - Creator
94. Latifjon - Kind and dear
95. Mansurali - Assisted by God
96. Nizom - Order, arrangement
97. Oyatulloh - Sign of God
98. Parvizjon - Happy and dear
99. Qudrat - Power, might
100. Rahmatulloh - Mercy of God

Kyrgyzstani baby names and their meanings

1. Adilet - justice
2. Aibek - moon master
3. Aigul - moon flower
4. Akylbek - wise master
5. Almaz - diamond
6. Altynai - golden moon
7. Anara - pomegranate
8. Arslan - lion
9. Asel - honey
10. Askar - soldier
11. Ayana - beautiful flower
12. Azat - free
13. Aziza - highly esteemed
14. Baktiyar - lucky
15. Begimai - princess
16. Bermet - pearl
17. Cholpon - Venus (morning star)
18. Damira - giving soul
19. Daniyar - wise
20. Dastan - story
21. Dinara - golden coin
22. Eldiyar - given by God
23. Elmira - princess
24. Emir - prince
25. Erkin - free
26. Farida - unique
27. Gulnara - pomegranate flower
28. Ilim - knowledge
29. Jamila - beautiful
30. Janyl - life
31. Kanat - wing
32. Kanykei - beloved wife
33. Kenesh - assembly
34. Kubanychbek - honored master

35. Kuralai - songbird
36. Kurmanbek - blessed master
37. Madina - city
38. Marat - desire
39. Meerim - kindness
40. Mirlan - lion
41. Nargiza - daffodil
42. Nasiba - destiny
43. Nurbek - light master
44. Nurlan - baby falcon
45. Oroz - fast
46. Raima - loving
47. Rakhat - comfort
48. Rysbek - brave master
49. Sabina - Sabine woman
50. Sabyr - patient
51. Sagyn - to praise
52. Salamat - health
53. Samat - support
54. Saniya - high, exalted
55. Shamil - comprehensive
56. Shyngys - conqueror
57. Sultan - ruler
58. Talant - talent
59. Tamara - palm tree
60. Tursunbek - blessed sun
61. Ulan - warrior
62. Urmat - desire
63. Umut - hope
64. Zere - gold
65. Zhyldyz - star
66. Aika - respect
67. Aiperi - moon beauty
68. Aisuluu - moon beauty
69. Almira - princess
70. Altyn - gold

71. Amina - trustworthy
72. Arzu - wish
73. Asan - easy
74. Aybek - moon master
75. Aziza - highly esteemed
76. Bakyt - happiness
77. Chynara - plane tree
78. Damir - heart
79. Dinar - gold coin
80. Elina - torch
81. Emir - commander
82. Erkin - free
83. Farida - precious
84. Gul - flower
85. Ilim - knowledge
86. Jamila - beautiful
87. Janyl - life
88. Kanat - wing
89. Kanykei - beloved wife
90. Kenesh - council
91. Kubanychbek - honored master
92. Kuralai - songbird
93. Kurmanbek - blessed master
94. Madina - city
95. Marat - desire
96. Meerim - kindness
97. Mirlan - lion
98. Nargiza - daffodil
99. Nasiba - destiny
100. Nurbek - light master

Turkmenistani baby names and their meanings

1. Abadan - Eternal
2. Aýberdi - Moon gave
3. Aýdogdy - Moon is born
4. Aýdogdymyrat - Moon-born wish
5. Aýjemal - Moon beauty
6. Aýnabat - Moon-like
7. Aýnagozel - Moon is beautiful
8. Aýnur - Moonlight
9. Aýşegul - Moon rose
10. Aýşem - Moon beauty
11. Babamyrat - Father's wish
12. Bagtyýar - Happy
13. Bahar - Spring
14. Baýram - Holiday
15. Baýramgül - Holiday flower
16. Baýrammyrat - Holiday wish
17. Begench - Joy
18. Begmyrat - Noble wish
19. Berdi - Gave
20. Berdymyrat - Given wish
21. Bilbil - Nightingale
22. Dilara - Heart's comfort
23. Döwlet - State, wealth
24. Döwletgeldi - State came
25. Döwletmämmet - State man
26. Döwletnazar - State sight
27. Döwletnur - State light
28. Döwran - Time, era
29. Enejan - Mother's soul
30. Eneýew - Mother's son
31. Ertir - Brave
32. Eýegözel - Eye beauty
33. Eýemämmet - Eye man

34. Eýemrat - Eye wish
35. Eýenur - Eye light
36. Gül - Flower
37. Gülbahar - Spring flower
38. Gülderen - Making smile
39. Güljamal - Flower beauty
40. Güljemal - Flower beauty
41. Gülşat - Flower garden
42. Günbatar - Sun is setting
43. Gündogar - East, sunrise
44. Günça - Sunflower
45. Günşat - Sun garden
46. Gurbangeldi - Hero came
47. Gurbannazar - Hero sight
48. Gurbansoltan - Hero sultan
49. Gurbanmyrat - Hero wish
50. Gurbannur - Hero light
51. Gülşenem - Flower beauty
52. Hydyr - Green, fresh
53. Ilaman - Fascinating
54. Ilgiz - Fascinate
55. Ilmyrat - Fascinating wish
56. Ilaman - Fascinating
57. Jahan - World
58. Jahanşat - World garden
59. Jahanmyrat - World wish
60. Jahanşah - World king
61. Jemile - Beauty
62. Jennet - Paradise
63. Jemal - Beauty
64. Kerim - Generous
65. Komek - Help
66. Komekgül - Help flower
67. Komeknazar - Help sight
68. Komekmyrat - Help wish
69. Komeknur - Help light

70. Mämmet - Man
71. Mämmetgeldi - Man came
72. Mämmetjan - Dear man
73. Mämmetmyrat - Man wish
74. Mämmetnazar - Man sight
75. Mämmetnur - Man light
76. Mähri - Kindness
77. Mähriban - Kind
78. Mährijemal - Kindness beauty
79. Mähriýew - Kind son
80. Mähriban - Kind
81. Mähri - Kindness
82. Mämmet - Man
83. Mähriban - Kind
84. Mämmetmyrat - Man wish
85. Mährijemal - Kindness beauty
86. Mähriýew - Kind son
87. Mähri - Kindness
88. Mämmet - Man
89. Mähriban - Kind
90. Mämmetmyrat - Man wish
91. Mährijemal - Kindness beauty
92. Mähriýew - Kind son
93. Mähri - Kindness
94. Mämmet - Man
95. Mähriban - Kind
96. Mämmetmyrat - Man wish
97. Mährijemal - Kindness beauty
98. Mähriýew - Kind son
99. Mähri - Kindness
100. Mämmet - Man

Mongolian baby names and their meanings

1. Altan - Golden
2. Batbayar - Strong joy
3. Bayarmaa - Mother of joy
4. Chuluun - Rock
5. Delger - Prosperous
6. Erdene - Jewel
7. Gantulga - Steel hearth
8. Gerel - Light
9. Hulan - Red fox
10. Jargal - Happiness
11. Khulan - Wild donkey
12. Munkh - Eternal
13. Narantsetseg - Sunflower
14. Oyun - Wisdom
15. Sarangerel - Moonlight
16. Togtokh - Durable
17. Uuganbayar - Happiness of dawn
18. Zorig - Brave
19. Batu - Loyal
20. Bolormaa - Crystal mother
21. Chimed - Immortal
22. Dulmaa - Lotus
23. Enkh - Peace
24. Ganbaatar - Steel hero
25. Ganzorig - Steel courage
26. Khongoroo - Camel
27. Munkhtsetseg - Eternal flower
28. Naran - Sun
29. Otgonbayar - Happiness of the west
30. Saruul - Agile
31. Tumur - Iron
32. Uyanga - Melody
33. Zolzaya - Beautiful fate
34. Bataa - Father

35. Chingis - Ocean
36. Enkhtuya - Ray of peace
37. Galbadrakh - Blessing
38. Khaliun - Gazelle
39. Munkhbat - Eternal firmness
40. Narangerel - Sunlight
41. Oyunchimeg - Wisdom ornament
42. Saran - Moon
43. Temuujin - Iron man
44. Uurtsaikh - Light of dawn
45. Zorigt - Brave man
46. Batkhuyag - Firm happiness
47. Delgertsetseg - Beautiful flower
48. Erdenechimeg - Jewel ornament
49. Gantugs - Steel flower
50. Khangai - Rich
51. Munkhtur - Eternal pillar
52. Naranbaatar - Sun hero
53. Otgontsetseg - Flower of the west
54. Sarantuya - Moonbeam
55. Tuvshintugs - Blessing of the light
56. Uyanga - Melody
57. Zolboo - Lucky
58. Batjargal - Firm happiness
59. Chuluunbaatar - Stone hero
60. Enkhjargal - Peaceful happiness
61. Galaa - Joy
62. Khurelbaatar - Wheel hero
63. Munkhbayar - Eternal joy
64. Narantuya - Sunbeam
65. Oyuunchimeg - Wisdom decoration
66. Saruultugs - Agile blessing
67. Tuya - Ray
68. Uugantsetseg - Dawn flower
69. Zolzaya - Beautiful fate
70. Batmunkh - Firm eternity

71. Delgermaa - Prosperous mother
72. Erdenebaatar - Jewel hero
73. Ganzul - Steel
74. Khulan - Onager
75. Munkhchimeg - Eternal decoration
76. Naranjargal - Sun happiness
77. Otgonjargal - Happiness of the west
78. Saruul - Agile
79. Tuvshinbayar - Blessing of the light
80. Uyanga - Melody
81. Zolbayar - Beautiful joy
82. Batu - Loyal
83. Chuluuntsetseg - Rock flower
84. Enkhtur - Ray of eternity
85. Galbadrakh - Blessing
86. Khongordzol - Camel fate
87. Munkhbayar - Eternal joy
88. Narantuya - Sunbeam
89. Oyuunchimeg - Wisdom decoration
90. Saranchimeg - Moon decoration
91. Tuya - Ray
92. Uuganaa - Dawn
93. Zoljargal - Beautiful happiness
94. Batkhuyag - Firm happiness
95. Delgerkhuyag - Prosperous happiness
96. Erdenechimeg - Jewel decoration
97. Gantulga - Steel hearth
98. Khulan - Onager
99. Munkhtuya - Eternal ray
100. Narangerel - Sunlight

Vietnamese baby names and their meanings

1. An - Peaceful
2. Bao - Protection
3. Chien - Fighter
4. Dung - Brave
5. Giang - River
6. Hien - Gentle, Nice
7. Khoa - Science, Knowledge
8. Long - Dragon
9. Minh - Bright
10. Nam - South
11. Phong - Wind
12. Quang - Clear, Bright
13. Sang - Noble, Upright
14. Tuan - Intelligent
15. Vu - Rain
16. Xuan - Spring
17. Yen - Peaceful, Calm
18. Binh - Peace
19. Cung - Bow, Arc
20. Dao - Peach Blossom
21. Duong - Virile
22. Hanh - Conduct, Behavior
23. Hoa - Flower
24. Kien - Persistent, Firm
25. Lam - Forest
26. Nghia - Righteous
27. Phuc - Blessing, Happiness
28. Quyen - Power, Right
29. Son - Mountain
30. Thanh - Clear, Pure
31. Trung - Loyal
32. Vinh - Glory
33. Thao - Respectful of Parents
34. Chi - Branch

35. Diep - Butterfly
36. Huyen - Black, Dark
37. Kim - Golden
38. Linh - Soul, Spirit
39. Mai - Cherry Blossom
40. Ngoc - Gem, Precious Stone
41. Phuong - Phoenix
42. Quy - Precious
43. Thu - Autumn
44. Trinh - Pure, Chaste
45. Xinh - Pretty, Beautiful
46. Lien - Lotus
47. Tuyet - Snow
48. Huong - Scent, Perfume
49. Thuy - Water
50. Nhung - Velvet
51. Anh - Intellect, Bright
52. Binh - Peaceful
53. Cuong - Strong, Healthy
54. Dinh - Palace, Camp
55. Huy - Glory, Honor
56. Khuong - Generous
57. Loc - Blessing, Favor
58. Nhan - Kind, Gentle
59. Phu - Wealthy
60. Quoc - Nation, Country
61. Tan - New
62. Truong - Long, Perpetual
63. Van - Literature, Culture
64. Thien - Heaven, Sky
65. Bach - White
66. Cong - Intelligent, Clever
67. Duy - Unique, Single
68. Hung - Brave, Heroic
69. Luan - Discussion, Debate
70. Nhat - Sun

71. Phuoc - Blessed, Lucky
72. Quan - Soldier, Warrior
73. Son - Mountain
74. Tung - Universal, General
75. Vuong - King
76. Thinh - Prosperous, Wealthy
77. Chau - Pearl, Gem
78. Dien - Crazy, Insane
79. Hoang - Yellow, Golden
80. Khanh - Celebration, Festival
81. Lan - Orchid
82. Ngan - Silver
83. Phong - Wind, Style
84. Quynh - A Type of Flower
85. Suong - Fog, Mist
86. Truc - Bamboo
87. Vien - Complete, Perfect
88. Thuy - Gentle, Nice
89. Bao - Treasure
90. Cuc - Chrysanthemum
91. Dong - Winter
92. Hao - Good, Perfect
93. Khiet - Pure, Clean
94. Lanh - Cold, Chilly
95. Ninh - Tranquil, Peaceful
96. Phuc - Blessing, Happiness
97. Quy - Precious, Valuable
98. Thang - Victory
99. Trong - Respectful, Reverent
100. Vu - Rain

Thai baby names and their meanings

1. Achara – Beautiful angel
2. Adithep – Lord of the sun
3. Aimon – Wealthy
4. Anuman – Small and mighty
5. Aroon – Dawn
6. Boonsri – Beautiful
7. Busarakham – Yellow sapphire
8. Chai – Victory
9. Chaiyan – Long life
10. Chalerm – Celebrated
11. Chanchai – Victorious
12. Charoen – Prosperous
13. Chatri – Brave knight
14. Darika – Star
15. Dara – Star
16. Duangkamol – From the heart
17. Fai – Fire
18. Fasai – Clear sky
19. Gaysorn – Crystal clear
20. Hansa – Supreme happiness
21. Inthira – Powerful
22. Itthi – Powerful
23. Jiraprapa – Glowing light
24. Kamon – Heart
25. Kanda – Beloved
26. Kanya – Young daughter
27. Kasem – Pure happiness
28. Kiet – Honored
29. Klahan – Brave
30. Kongdej – Victory
31. Kraisorn – Proud
32. Krung – City
33. Ladda – Beautiful woman
34. Lalida – Adorable person

35. Lamai – Gentle
36. Lawan – Beautiful
37. Lek – Small
38. Malee – Jasmine flower
39. Manop – Bird
40. Nanda – Prosperous
41. Niran – Eternal
42. Nit – Angel
43. Nok – Bird
44. Nuan – Warm
45. Pan – Leaf
46. Panya – Knowledge
47. Pichai – Victorious
48. Pim – Strange
49. Ploy – Gemstone
50. Prasert – Excellent
51. Ratri – Night
52. Ratree – Night flower
53. Rung – Rainbow
54. Saengdao – Starlight
55. Saichon – Peaceful life
56. Sakda – Power
57. Samorn – Beautiful and beloved
58. Sanoh – Sweet and pleasant
59. Saran – Joy
60. Sarit – Diamond
61. Somchai – Man of worth
62. Somwang – Hopeful
63. Songkran – Water festival
64. Suda – Noble
65. Sudarat – Beautiful lady
66. Suk – Happiness
67. Sukhon – Fragrance
68. Sunan – Good word
69. Suphannika – Golden lady
70. Sutat – Excellent

71. Suthida – Good luck
72. Tawee – Large
73. Thaksin – South
74. Than – Million
75. Thara – Wealth
76. Thip – Angel
77. Thong – Gold
78. Thongchai – Golden victory
79. Udom – The best
80. Urai – Water
81. Vasana – Scent
82. Virote – Great
83. Wann – Sweet
84. Wannika – Beautiful angel
85. Wari – Rose
86. Wasana – Luck
87. Wimon – Ring
88. Wisit – Clear
89. Yindee – Pleasure
90. Ying – Female
91. Yod – Excellent
92. Yuth – Fight
93. Boon-Nam – Born with good fortune
94. Chalad – Smart
95. Daeng – Red
96. Ekachai – Victorious
97. Faasai – Clear sky
98. Kallaya – Beautiful, good
99. Lawana – Beautiful
100. Malai – Garland of flowers

Malaysian baby names and their meanings

1. Aiman - lucky, blessed
2. Adira - strong, noble
3. Afiq - honest, upright
4. Batrisyia - intelligent, wise
5. Balqis - name of the Queen of Sheba
6. Cempaka - a type of flower
7. Dania - close, near
8. Ehsan - charity, compassion
9. Fadil - generous, honorable
10. Farah - joy, happiness
11. Ghazi - warrior, conqueror
12. Hana - happiness, bliss
13. Iman - faith, belief
14. Jasmin - a type of flower
15. Kamil - perfect, complete
16. Laila - night, dark beauty
17. Malik - king, sovereign
18. Nadia - caller, announcer
19. Omar - flourishing, long-lived
20. Putri - princess
21. Qasim - distributor, divider
22. Rafiq - friend, companion
23. Syafiq - compassionate, kind
24. Tariq - morning star
25. Umar - life, long living
26. Vania - butterfly
27. Wahid - unique, singular
28. Yasmin - jasmine flower
29. Zafir - victorious, successful
30. Aida - visitor, returning
31. Budi - wisdom, mind
32. Cahaya - light, radiance
33. Daud - beloved, friend
34. Elina - intelligent, bright

35. Fazil - virtuous, superior
36. Ghani - rich, wealthy
37. Hafiz - guardian, protector
38. Izzat - honor, prestige
39. Jannah - paradise, heaven
40. Khalid - eternal, immortal
41. Lutfi - kind, gentle
42. Malaika - angels
43. Nabil - noble, generous
44. Othman - companion, friend
45. Putra - son, prince
46. Qadir - capable, powerful
47. Rafi - exalted, sublime
48. Syed - noble, respected
49. Tahir - pure, clean
50. Uzma - greatest, supreme
51. Vivi - alive, lively
52. Wafi - faithful, loyal
53. Yamin - right, proper
54. Zaim - leader, chief
55. Afiqah - honest, upright
56. Badri - full moon
57. Camelia - a type of flower
58. Danish - knowledge, wisdom
59. Ezzah - respect, honor
60. Fatin - captivating, alluring
61. Ghazali - mystic, philosopher
62. Hidayah - guidance, instruction
63. Iskandar - defender, helper
64. Jazmin - jasmine flower
65. Kamal - perfection, integrity
66. Latif - gentle, kind
67. Marwan - solid, strong
68. Najwa - secret, whisper
69. Omar - flourishing, long-lived
70. Puteri - princess, daughter

71. Qamar - moon, satellite
72. Rasyid - rightly guided
73. Syahmi - famous, renowned
74. Taufiq - successful, prosperous
75. Ummi - my mother
76. Vina - lute, stringed instrument
77. Wajih - noble, honored
78. Yasir - wealthy, prosperous
79. Zahir - bright, shining
80. Aqil - intelligent, wise
81. Batrisya - intelligent, wise
82. Cinta - love, affection
83. Dian - candle, light
84. Elma - apple
85. Fadhil - generous, honorable
86. Ghaida - soft, gentle
87. Hani - happy, delighted
88. Irfan - knowledge, learning
89. Jafar - small stream
90. Khalifah - successor, steward
91. Lina - tender, delicate
92. Mahir - skilled, expert
93. Naim - comfort, tranquility
94. Osman - servant of God
95. Putra - son, prince
96. Qais - firm, hard
97. Rafidah - support, prop
98. Syakir - thankful, grateful
99. Tasya - resurrection
100. Umar - life, long living

Indonesian baby names and their meanings

1. Aditya – The Sun
2. Agus – Good, Excellent
3. Aisyah – Life, Vivaciousness
4. Ajeng – Respectful
5. Akbar – Great
6. Alif – First Character in Arabic
7. Amalia – Industrious, Striving
8. Andi – Warrior
9. Anggun – Graceful
10. Aninda – Dear, Beloved
11. Anwar – Bright
12. Ari – Lion
13. Arjuna – Bright, Shining
14. Arya – Noble
15. Asmara – Love, Romance
16. Ayu – Beautiful
17. Bagus – Handsome, Good
18. Bambang – Knight
19. Bayu – Wind
20. Bella – Beautiful
21. Bintang – Star
22. Budi – Reason, Mind
23. Cahya – Light, Radiance
24. Candra – Moon
25. Cinta – Love
26. Dara – Virgin, Maiden
27. Daud – Beloved
28. Dewi – Goddess
29. Dian – Candle, Light
30. Eka – First
31. Endah – Beautiful
32. Fajar – Dawn
33. Farah – Joy, Happiness
34. Fitri – Pure

35. Galih – Jade, Precious Stone
36. Garuda – Mythical Bird
37. Gita – Song
38. Hadi – Leader, Guide
39. Hanif – True, Upright
40. Harun – Mountain
41. Hasan – Handsome, Good
42. Hidayat – Guidance
43. Ika – One
44. Indah – Beautiful
45. Irfan – Knowledge, Learning
46. Iskandar – Defender of Mankind
47. Jaya – Victorious
48. Kadek – Younger Sibling
49. Kusuma – Flower
50. Lestari – Eternal, Everlasting
51. Lia – Guardian, Protector
52. Lintang – Star
53. Made – Mother
54. Mahesa – Great
55. Malik – King
56. Mawar – Rose
57. Maya – Illusion, Magic
58. Mega – Cloud
59. Melati – Jasmine Flower
60. Nia – Purpose
61. Nila – Blue
62. Ningsih – Love
63. Nisa – Women
64. Nur – Light
65. Pertiwi – Earth
66. Prabu – King
67. Putra – Son
68. Putri – Daughter
69. Raka – Full Moon
70. Rani – Queen

71. Ratna – Jewel
72. Reza – Contentment
73. Rizki – Blessing
74. Sari – Essence
75. Satria – Knight, Warrior
76. Septi – Seventh
77. Sinta – Love
78. Siti – Lady, Woman
79. Surya – Sun
80. Tari – Dance
81. Tegar – Firm, Steadfast
82. Tia – Princess
83. Tirta – Holy Water
84. Ujang – Boy
85. Utari – Morning
86. Vania – Butterfly
87. Wati – Female
88. Wira – Hero
89. Wisnu – Preserver
90. Yanti – Beautiful
91. Yudha – Warrior
92. Yuni – Beautiful
93. Zahra – Flower, Blossom
94. Zaki – Pure
95. Zara – Princess
96. Zulaikha – Brilliant Beauty
97. Suryani – Sunshine
98. Dewantara – King of Gods
99. Purnama – Full Moon
100. Adinda – Younger Sister

Filipino baby names and their meanings

1. Adela – Noble
2. Agnes – Pure
3. Alon – Wave
4. Amihan – Northeast wind
5. Antonio – Priceless
6. Arsenio – Masculine, virile
7. Arturo – Bear
8. Aurora – Dawn
9. Bayani – Hero
10. Beatriz – Bringer of Joy
11. Benigno – Kind
12. Buenaventura – Good fortune
13. Cesar – Long-haired
14. Consuelo – Comfort
15. Corazon – Heart
16. Dalisay – Pure
17. Danilo – God is my judge
18. Darna – A stone
19. Delia – Person from Delos
20. Diwa – Spirit
21. Dolores – Sorrows
22. Eduardo – Wealthy guardian
23. Elpidio – Hope
24. Erlinda – Tender and beautiful
25. Esperanza – Hope
26. Estrella – Star
27. Eugenio – Well-born
28. Fe – Faith
29. Fernando – Adventurous
30. Florante – Blooming
31. Francisco – Free
32. Gabriela – God is my strength
33. Gloria – Glory
34. Gregorio – Watchful

35. Halina – Come
36. Hector – To hold
37. Imelda – Warrior woman
38. Isagani – Prosperous
39. Isko – God is gracious
40. Jaime – Supplanter
41. Javier – Bright
42. Jesusa – God is salvation
43. Jose – He will add
44. Juan – God is gracious
45. Juana – God is gracious
46. Julio – Youthful
47. Luningning – Brightness
48. Ma Theresa – Bitter harvester
49. Magdalena – Woman from Magdala
50. Manuel – God is with us
51. Marcelo – Little warrior
52. Maria – Bitter
53. Mariano – Male
54. Maricar – Bitter beloved
55. Mario – Male
56. Mayumi – True gentle beauty
57. Milagros – Miracles
58. Nenita – Little girl
59. Norma – Rule
60. Pacita – Peaceful
61. Paloma – Dove
62. Pilar – Pillar
63. Ramon – Wise protector
64. Raquel – Ewe
65. Renato – Reborn
66. Ricardo – Brave ruler
67. Roberto – Bright fame
68. Rodel – Famous ruler
69. Rodrigo – Famous ruler
70. Rolando – Famous throughout the land

71. Rosalinda – Beautiful rose
72. Rosario – Rosary
73. Salvador – Savior
74. Santiago – Saint James
75. Santos – Saints
76. Sergio – Servant
77. Socorro – Help
78. Soledad – Solitude
79. Susana – Lily
80. Tala – Star
81. Teresa – Harvester
82. Trinidad – Trinity
83. Vicente – Conquering
84. Victoria – Victory
85. Virgilio – Flourishing
86. Zenaida – Life of Zeus
87. Lualhati – Peace and tranquility
88. Ligaya – Joy
89. Malaya – Free
90. Harana – Serenade
91. Mabuhay – Long live
92. Mahal – Love
93. Mutya – Pearl
94. Mayari – Moon goddess
95. Diwata – Fairy
96. Lakan – Noble man
97. Lakambini – Lady of importance
98. Panday – Blacksmith
99. Bagani – Warrior
100. Sinta – Beloved

Singaporean baby names and their meanings

1. Aiden - Fiery one
2. Adeline - Noble and kind
3. Ai - Love and affection
4. Alvin - Wise friend
5. Amelia - Industrious, striving
6. Benjamin - Son of the right hand
7. Brandon - Prince, or brave
8. Chloe - Blooming, fertility
9. Darren - Great
10. Emily - Industrious, striving
11. Ethan - Strong, firm
12. Felicia - Happy, lucky
13. Gabriel - God is my strength
14. Hannah - Grace, favor
15. Ivan - God is gracious
16. Jasmine - Gift from God, flower
17. Kai - Ocean or restoration
18. Li - Beautiful, powerful
19. Marcus - Warlike, Mars
20. Naomi - Pleasantness
21. Oliver - Olive tree
22. Patricia - Noble, patrician
23. Quentin - Fifth
24. Rachel - Ewe, sheep
25. Samuel - God has heard
26. Tiffany - God's appearance
27. Uriel - God is my light
28. Victoria - Victory
29. William - Resolute protector
30. Xander - Defender of the people
31. Yvonne - Yew, archer
32. Zachary - Remembered by God
33. Ariel - Lion of God

34. Beatrice - She who makes happy
35. Calvin - Bald, hairless
36. Doris - Gift
37. Edwin - Wealthy friend
38. Fiona - Fair, white, beautiful
39. Gerald - Rule of the spear
40. Heidi - Noble, kind
41. Iris - Rainbow
42. Justin - Just, fair
43. Kimberly - From the wood of the royal forest
44. Lawrence - From Laurentum
45. Monica - Advisor
46. Nigel - Champion
47. Opal - Jewel
48. Priscilla - Ancient
49. Ronald - Ruler's counselor
50. Sylvia - From the forest
51. Travis - To cross over
52. Ursula - Little bear
53. Vanessa - Butterfly
54. Wayne - Wagon maker
55. Xavier - The new house
56. Yolanda - Violet flower
57. Zane - God is gracious
58. Adele - Noble, kind
59. Bernard - Brave as a bear
60. Cindy - Moon
61. Derek - People's ruler
62. Elaine - Light
63. Frederick - Peaceful ruler
64. Grace - God's favor
65. Howard - High guardian
66. Isabelle - God is my oath
67. Jackson - Son of Jack
68. Linda - Pretty
69. Maxwell - Great stream

70. Nancy - Grace
71. Oscar - God's spear
72. Penelope - Weaver
73. Quincy - Fifth
74. Rebecca - To bind
75. Stanley - Stony meadow
76. Theresa - Summer, harvest
77. Ulysses - Wrathful
78. Valerie - Strength, health
79. Wendy - Wanderer
80. Xavier - New house
81. Yvette - Yew, archer
82. Zoe - Life
83. Audrey - Noble strength
84. Bradley - Broad meadow
85. Charlotte - Free man
86. Damian - To tame
87. Eunice - Good victory
88. Franklin - Free man
89. Glenda - Holy and good
90. Harold - Army ruler
91. Irene - Peace
92. Jasper - Treasurer
93. Kendra - Understanding
94. Leonard - Lion strength
95. Meredith - Great lord
96. Norma - Rule, norm
97. Octavia - Eighth
98. Phoebe - Bright, pure
99. Rupert - Bright fame
100. Serena - Tranquil, serene

Cambodian baby names and their meanings

1. Achariya - Miraculous
2. Bopha - Flower
3. Chanda - Heart
4. Dara - Star
5. Eang - Bright
6. Fane - Free spirit
7. Gita - Song
8. Heng - Fortunate
9. Indira - Beauty
10. Jaya - Victory
11. Kalyan - Welfare
12. Lina - Tender
13. Maly - Flower
14. Nanda - Joy
15. Oudom - Superior
16. Pisey - Lovely
17. Quy - Precious
18. Rithy - Power
19. Sopheap - Gentle
20. Thida - Daughter
21. Udom - Lucky
22. Vanna - Golden
23. Watey - Peaceful
24. Xomphi - Blessed
25. Yuth - Justice
26. Zalika - Well born
27. Amara - Immortal
28. Bora - Excellent
29. Chhay - Shadow
30. Dany - God is my judge
31. Eath - Grandfather
32. Fai - Sky
33. Gita - Song
34. Hani - Happy

35. Indra - God of rain and thunder
36. Jorani - Radiant jewel
37. Kiri - Mountain
38. Lida - Loved by everyone
39. Mina - Love
40. Nary - Woman
41. Oudom - Superior
42. Pich - Diamond
43. Quan - Bright
44. Rith - Light
45. Soriya - Sun
46. Theara - Angel
47. Uy - Jade
48. Vichea - Wisdom
49. Wath - Time
50. Xanthe - Golden
51. Yos - Fame
52. Zola - Peaceful
53. Arun - Sun
54. Bopha - Flower
55. Chhaya - Shadow
56. Dara - Star
57. Eang - Bright
58. Fane - Free spirit
59. Gita - Song
60. Heng - Fortunate
61. Indira - Beauty
62. Jaya - Victory
63. Kalyan - Welfare
64. Lina - Tender
65. Maly - Flower
66. Nanda - Joy
67. Oudom - Superior
68. Pisey - Lovely
69. Quy - Precious
70. Rithy - Power

71. Sopheap - Gentle
72. Thida - Daughter
73. Udom - Lucky
74. Vanna - Golden
75. Watey - Peaceful
76. Xomphi - Blessed
77. Yuth - Justice
78. Zalika - Well born
79. Amara - Immortal
80. Bora - Excellent
81. Chhay - Shadow
82. Dany - God is my judge
83. Eath - Grandfather
84. Fai - Sky
85. Gita - Song
86. Hani - Happy
87. Indra - God of rain and thunder
88. Jorani - Radiant jewel
89. Kiri - Mountain
90. Lida - Loved by everyone
91. Mina - Love
92. Nary - Woman
93. Oudom - Superior
94. Pich - Diamond
95. Quan - Bright
96. Rith - Light
97. Soriya - Sun
98. Theara - Angel
99. Uy - Jade
100. Vichea - Wisdom

Laotian baby names and their meanings

1. Achariya - miracle
2. Aksone - celebration
3. Bounmy - good fortune
4. Bounthanh - worthwhile life
5. Chanda - beloved
6. Chanthaly - moon-faced girl
7. Dalavone - beautiful moon
8. Darasavanh - star in the sky
9. Dara - star
10. Fasai - clear sky
11. Inthira - goddess of the sky
12. Kanya - girl
13. Khamla - golden
14. Khampheng - strong
15. Khamsouk - golden flower
16. Khanthaly - precious garland
17. Khouanfa - heavenly aroma
18. Lanxang - million elephants
19. Latsamy - sweet and charming
20. Latsavong - righteous life
21. Malyna - little blossom
22. Manisone - beautiful gem
23. Naly - lovely
24. Nang - lady
25. Nini - delicate
26. Nouda - little rice stalk
27. Oula - precious jade
28. Phaivanh - glorious life
29. Phet - diamond
30. Phonethip - artistic
31. Phoudoi - mountain
32. Phouma - fortunate
33. Phousavanh - paradise
34. Saengdao - starlight

35. Saengmany - fortunate light
36. Saengphet - diamond light
37. Saengphone - gift of light
38. Saengsavan - golden light
39. Saengsen - magical light
40. Saengtawan - light of dawn
41. Sengdao - path of the stars
42. Sengmany - blessed light
43. Sengsavane - golden light
44. Sengsay - voice of light
45. Sivilay - beautiful creation
46. Somchit - fortunate
47. Somphone - golden gift
48. Somphou - gifted one
49. Souk - market
50. Soukphaly - successful market
51. Souksavanh - happy market
52. Sounantha - heavenly sound
53. Soutchai - victory
54. Thavone - fortunate star
55. Thipphay - celestial nymph
56. Thongbay - golden silk
57. Vanida - girl
58. Vanleng - sweet voice
59. Vannasone - beautiful sound
60. Vannavong - long life
61. Vatsana - rain
62. Viengkham - golden city
63. Viengsavanh - paradise city
64. Xay - victory
65. Xaysana - victorious rain
66. Xayvong - victorious life
67. Xoumphon - blessed gift
68. Xoumphonphakdy - blessed gift of victory
69. Boun - merit
70. Bounthavy - merit and prosperity

71. Chanh - moon
72. Chanthavong - long life
73. Chansavang - golden moon
74. Daovone - beautiful moon
75. Fasai - clear sky
76. Inthavong - king of heaven
77. Kham - gold
78. Khamhoung - golden swan
79. Khampheng - strong
80. Khamvongsa - golden bird
81. Khamsouk - golden flower
82. Khan - prince
83. Khanthavong - long life
84. Khonesavanh - golden star
85. Latsamy - sweet and charming
86. Latsavong - righteous life
87. Manola - beautiful ruby
88. Nouda - little rice stalk
89. Phaeng - diamond
90. Phet - diamond
91. Phonethip - artistic
92. Phoudoi - mountain
93. Phouma - fortunate
94. Saeng - light
95. Saengdao - starlight
96. Saengphet - diamond light
97. Saengphone - gift of light
98. Sivilay - beautiful creation
99. Somphone - golden gift
100. Souk - market

Bruneian baby names and their meanings

1. Abdullah – Servant of God
2. Afiq – Honest, trustworthy
3. Aiman – Lucky, on the right
4. Akmal – Perfect, complete
5. Alif – Friendly, sociable
6. Amir – Prince, leader
7. Anis – Friendly, close friend
8. Arif – Knowledgeable, wise
9. Azim – Determined, resolved
10. Badrul – Full moon
11. Bahar – Spring, prime of life
12. Basir – One who sees, observer
13. Daud – Beloved, dear
14. Ehsan – Charitable, compassionate
15. Fadil – Generous, honorable
16. Ghazi – Warrior, conqueror
17. Hakim – Wise, judicious
18. Hamid – Praiseworthy, commendable
19. Idris – Studious, learned
20. Irfan – Knowledge, awareness
21. Jalil – Great, revered
22. Kamal – Perfection, completeness
23. Latif – Gentle, kind
24. Malik – King, ruler
25. Nadim – Friend, companion
26. Naim – Comfort, tranquility
27. Omar – Life, long living
28. Qasim – Divider, distributor
29. Rafiq – Friend, companion
30. Saif – Sword, bravery
31. Taufiq – Success, fortune
32. Umar – Life, long living
33. Wafi – Faithful, loyal
34. Yahya – God is gracious

35. Zahir – Bright, shining
36. Aida – Reward, present
37. Aisyah – Alive, well
38. Amira – Princess, leader
39. Aziza – Precious, cherished
40. Badriyah – Resembling the full moon
41. Dalia – Gentle, slender
42. Fatima – Captivating, charming
43. Ghazala – Deer, graceful
44. Hana – Happiness, bliss
45. Iman – Faith, belief
46. Jamila – Beautiful, attractive
47. Khalida – Eternal, everlasting
48. Laila – Night, dark beauty
49. Mariam – Sea of bitterness, rebelliousness
50. Nadia – Caller, announcer
51. Nura – Light, radiance
52. Qamar – Moon, satellite
53. Rabia – Spring, springtime
54. Saba – Morning, dawn
55. Tahira – Pure, chaste
56. Uzma – Greatest, more supreme
57. Widad – Love, friendship
58. Yasmin – Jasmine flower
59. Zahra – Flower, beauty
60. Aqil – Intelligent, wise
61. Bari – Creator, maker
62. Dzul – Possessor, owner
63. Fauzi – Successful, victorious
64. Hakimi – Judge, ruler
65. Ikhwan – Brotherhood, fraternity
66. Jalal – Majesty, grandeur
67. Kamali – Perfection, integrity
68. Latiff – Gentle, kind
69. Malik – King, ruler
70. Nadhir – Warner, herald

71. Naim – Comfort, tranquility
72. Omar – Life, long living
73. Qadir – Capable, powerful
74. Rafi – High, exalted
75. Saifuddin – Sword of the faith
76. Taufik – Successful, fortunate
77. Umar – Life, long living
78. Wafiq – Successful, victorious
79. Yahya – God is gracious
80. Zahid – Ascetic, devotee
81. Aini – Spring, well
82. Aisyah – Alive, well
83. Amalia – Industrious, striving
84. Azura – Sky blue
85. Badriyah – Resembling the full moon
86. Dalila – Gentle, kind
87. Fatimah – Captivating, charming
88. Ghazali – Deer, gazelle
89. Hani – Happy, delighted
90. Imani – Faith, belief
91. Jamilah – Beautiful, attractive
92. Khalilah – Friend, companion
93. Laila – Night, dark beauty
94. Mariam – Sea of bitterness, rebelliousness
95. Nadia – Caller, announcer
96. Nura – Light, radiance
97. Qamari – Moonlit, luminous
98. Rabiah – Spring, springtime
99. Sabah – Morning, dawn
100. Tahira – Pure, chaste

Taiwanese baby names and their meanings

1. Ai - love or affection
2. An - peace or tranquility
3. Bao - treasure or precious
4. Chao - exceeding or surpass
5. Chen - dawn or break of day
6. Cheng - become or succeed
7. Da - achieve or victory
8. Ding - decide or settle
9. En - kindness or charity
10. Fan - ordinary or normal
11. Fei - fly or soar
12. Feng - wind or breeze
13. Gang - strong or healthy
14. Gui - honorable or respectable
15. Hai - sea or ocean
16. Han - brave or heroic
17. Hong - wild swan or great
18. Hua - flower or blossom
19. Hui - bright or intelligent
20. Jian - healthy or strong
21. Jie - clean or pure
22. Jing - quiet or still
23. Kang - health or well-being
24. Lei - thunder or storm
25. Li - beautiful or pretty
26. Ling - spirit or soul
27. Min - quick or clever
28. Ming - bright or light
29. Nan - south or male
30. Ping - peace or level
31. Qiang - strong or powerful
32. Qiu - autumn or fall
33. Rong - glory or honor
34. Shan - mountain or hill

35. Shui - water or river
36. Tai - great or extreme
37. Tao - peach or long life
38. Ting - listen or hear
39. Wei - power or high
40. Xiang - good luck or auspicious
41. Xiao - morning or bright
42. Xin - new or fresh
43. Xue - snow or learning
44. Yan - beautiful or graceful
45. Ying - brave or hero
46. Yong - brave or forever
47. Yue - moon or music
48. Zhen - precious or valuable
49. Zhong - loyal or faithful
50. Zi - son or child
51. An-Ping - peaceful or tranquil
52. Bi-Ling - jasmine bell
53. Chao-Xing - morning star
54. Da-Xia - big hero
55. En-Lai - favor coming
56. Fang-Yu - fragrant jade
57. Guo-Hui - country's wisdom
58. Heng-Yi - persistent righteousness
59. Jian-Min - healthy and clever
60. Kang-Da - healthy and big
61. Li-Hua - pear blossom
62. Min-Jie - quick and pure
63. Nan-Feng - south wind
64. Pei-Ying - jade brightness
65. Qiu-Ling - autumn spirit
66. Rui-Li - intelligent and beautiful
67. Shan-Hai - mountain and sea
68. Ting-Feng - listen to the wind
69. Wei-Ming - great brightness
70. Xiang-Li - good luck and beautiful

71. Xiao-Ling - morning spirit
72. Yan-Ping - peaceful swallow
73. Zhen-Zhen - precious and valuable
74. Ai-Ling - love spirit
75. Bei-Bei - precious jade
76. Cheng-Han - successful and heroic
77. Duo-Duo - much much
78. En-Pei - graceful jade
79. Feng-Mian - wind and cotton
80. Guo-Jian - country's health
81. Hui-Ming - bright wisdom
82. Jian-Ying - healthy and heroic
83. Kang-Li - healthy and beautiful
84. Li-Ming - beautiful light
85. Min-Feng - clever wind
86. Nan-Hai - south sea
87. Pei-Ling - jade spirit
88. Qiu-Yue - autumn moon
89. Rui-Feng - intelligent wind
90. Shan-Li - mountain beauty
91. Ting-Hai - listen to the sea
92. Wei-Ping - great peace
93. Xiang-Min - good luck and cleverness
94. Xiao-Mei - morning beauty
95. Yan-Rong - beautiful glory
96. Zhen-Li - precious beauty
97. Ai-Mei - love beauty
98. Bei-Feng - precious wind
99. Cheng-Li - successful beauty
100. Duo-Li - much beauty

Hong Kong baby names and their meanings

1. Aiden – fiery
2. Ava – like a bird
3. Brian – strong, virtuous, and honorable
4. Chloe – blooming
5. Ethan – strong and enduring
6. Emily – industrious
7. Felix – happy and lucky
8. Grace – gracious
9. Henry – ruler of the home
10. Isabella – pledged to God
11. Jack – God is gracious
12. Kaitlyn – pure
13. Liam – strong-willed warrior
14. Mia – mine
15. Noah – comfort and rest
16. Olivia – olive tree
17. Patrick – nobleman
18. Quinn – wisdom, reason
19. Ryan – little king
20. Sophia – wisdom
21. Tyler – tile maker
22. Victoria – victory
23. William – resolute protection
24. Zoe – life
25. Aaron – high mountain
26. Bella – beautiful
27. Charles – free man
28. Daisy – day's eye
29. Edward – rich guard
30. Fiona – white, fair
31. George – farmer
32. Hannah – grace
33. Ian – God is gracious
34. Jasmine – gift from God

35. Kevin – handsome
36. Lily – lily flower
37. Matthew – gift of God
38. Natalie – birthday of the Lord
39. Oscar – deer friend
40. Penelope – weaver
41. Raymond – wise protector
42. Stella – star
43. Timothy – honoring God
44. Ursula – little bear
45. Vincent – conquering
46. Wendy – friend
47. Xavier – the new house
48. Yvonne – yew wood
49. Zachary – remembered by God
50. Amy – beloved
51. Bruce – from the brushwood thicket
52. Cindy – moon
53. Daniel – God is my judge
54. Emma – universal
55. Frank – free man
56. Gloria – glory
57. Howard – high guardian
58. Ivy – faithfulness
59. Justin – just, fair
60. Kimberly – from the royal fortress meadow
61. Lawrence – from Laurentum
62. Monica – advisor
63. Norman – northerner
64. Octavia – eighth
65. Peter – rock
66. Queenie – queen's woman
67. Ronald – ruler's counselor
68. Samantha – listener
69. Terry – power of the tribe
70. Ursula – little bear

71. Veronica – true image
72. Walter – ruler of the army
73. Xander – defending men
74. Yolanda – violet flower
75. Zara – princess
76. Albert – noble, bright
77. Brenda – sword
78. Calvin – bald
79. Doris – gift
80. Elvis – all wise
81. Flora – flower
82. Gregory – watchful, alert
83. Iris – rainbow
84. Jerome – sacred name
85. Karen – pure
86. Leonard – lion strength
87. Miranda – worthy of admiration
88. Nigel – dark night
89. Opal – jewel
90. Priscilla – ancient
91. Quentin – fifth
92. Rita – pearl
93. Stanley – near the stony clearing
94. Teresa – harvest
95. Ulysses – wrathful
96. Vanessa – butterfly
97. Wallace – foreigner
98. Xena – guest, stranger
99. Yvette – yew
100. Zephyr – west wind

Macau baby names and their meanings

1. Aiden – little fire
2. Aimee – beloved
3. Alvin – noble friend
4. Amara – grace
5. Angela – messenger of God
6. Anson – son of Ann
7. Ava – life
8. Benjamin – son of the right hand
9. Bella – beautiful
10. Brian – strong, virtuous
11. Caleb – faithful
12. Chloe – blooming
13. Damian – to tame
14. Danielle – God is my judge
15. Edward – wealthy guardian
16. Elise – pledged to God
17. Ethan – strong, firm
18. Fiona – white, fair
19. Gabriel – God is my strength
20. Grace – grace
21. Henry – ruler of the home
22. Isabella – pledged to God
23. Jack – God is gracious
24. Jade – precious stone
25. Kai – sea
26. Kaitlyn – pure
27. Leo – lion
28. Lily – lily flower
29. Lucas – light
30. Madison – son of Maud
31. Nathan – gift from God
32. Olivia – olive tree
33. Patrick – nobleman
34. Penelope – weaver

35. Quentin – fifth
36. Rachel – ewe
37. Samuel – God has heard
38. Sophia – wisdom
39. Thomas – twin
40. Victoria – victory
41. William – resolute protector
42. Xavier – bright, splendid
43. Zachary – God has remembered
44. Zoe – life
45. Adrian – sea or water
46. Beatrice – bringer of joy
47. Carmen – song
48. Derek – ruler of the people
49. Emily – rival
50. Francis – free man
51. Gerald – ruler with the spear
52. Helen – bright, shining one
53. Ivan – God is gracious
54. Jasmine – jasmine flower
55. Kevin – handsome
56. Laura – laurel
57. Marcus – warlike
58. Nicole – victory of the people
59. Oscar – deer friend
60. Paula – small
61. Raymond – wise protector
62. Serena – serene, calm
63. Timothy – honoring God
64. Ursula – little bear
65. Vincent – conqueror
66. Wendy – wanderer
67. Yvonne – yew wood
68. Zoe – life
69. Aaron – high mountain
70. Bernadette – brave as a bear

71. Charles – free man
72. Daphne – laurel tree
73. Eugene – well-born
74. Felicity – happiness
75. George – farmer
76. Hazel – hazelnut tree
77. Iris – rainbow
78. Justin – just, fair
79. Kimberly – from the royal fortress meadow
80. Leonard – brave lion
81. Monica – advisor
82. Nigel – dark, black
83. Opal – jewel
84. Phoebe – bright, pure
85. Ronald – ruler's counselor
86. Stella – star
87. Terrence – tender, gracious
88. Ursula – little bear
89. Vivian – alive
90. Wallace – foreigner
91. Xander – defending men
92. Yolanda – violet flower
93. Zara – princess
94. Abel – breath
95. Bianca – white
96. Clifford – ford by a cliff
97. Delilah – delicate
98. Ernest – serious, resolute
99. Fabian – bean grower
100. Giselle – pledge

Tibetan baby names and their meanings

1. Tenzin - Protector of the teachings of Buddha
2. Lhamo - Goddess
3. Pema - Lotus
4. Sonam - Merit
5. Dorje - Indestructible
6. Kunchok - Rare Jewel
7. Jigme - Fearless
8. Rinchen - Precious Jewel
9. Choden - One who is devout
10. Norbu - Jewel
11. Paljor - Glorious
12. Dechen - Great Bliss
13. Chimi - Immortal
14. Tashi - Auspicious
15. Tsomo - Lake
16. Namgyal - Victorious in all directions
17. Lobsang - Mind of Enlightenment
18. Karma - Action
19. Dawa - Moon
20. Ngawang - Power of Speech
21. Rigzin - Holder of the lineage
22. Tsering - Long Life
23. Wangchuk - Mighty
24. Thubten - Buddha's teachings
25. Yonten - Knowledgeable
26. Sangay - Buddha
27. Palden - Glorious
28. Kalden - Golden Age
29. Jamyang - Gentle Voice
30. Trinley - Buddha's activities
31. Gyatso - Ocean
32. Sherab - Wisdom
33. Chogden - Supreme Dharma
34. Tseten - Firm Life

35. Champa - Love
36. Gyaltsen - Victory Banner
37. Samdup - Fulfillment of Wishes
38. Yangchen - Melodious Voice
39. Yeshe - Wisdom
40. Drolma - Female Buddha
41. Wangmo - Powerful Lady
42. Dakpa - Brave
43. Tsultrim - Ethical Discipline
44. Gyurme - Everlasting
45. Drakpa - Bold
46. Tashi - Good Luck
47. Choying - Dharma Melody
48. Tsewang - Long Life
49. Pasang - Born on a Friday
50. Zopa - Patience
51. Selden - Clear Mind
52. Jampa - Loving Kindness
53. Diki - Healthy and Wealthy
54. Thinley - Ethical Actions
55. Lhundup - Spontaneously Accomplished
56. Choedon - Dharma Lamp
57. Tsundue - Conscientious
58. Kunga - Good Fortune
59. Delek - Happiness and Prosperity
60. Phuntsok - Spontaneous Perfection
61. Pelden - Glorious
62. Thrinley - Fruitful Action
63. Chophel - Dharma Flourishing
64. Tenzing - Upholder of Teachings
65. Gyurmed - Eternal
66. Tsering - Long Life
67. Yeshi - Wisdom
68. Tashi - Auspicious
69. Pema - Lotus
70. Sonam - Merit

71. Wangyal - Power
72. Dawa - Moon
73. Lhamo - Goddess
74. Kelsang - Good Fortune
75. Tsomo - Lake
76. Jigme - Fearless
77. Norbu - Jewel
78. Choden - Devout
79. Rinchen - Precious Jewel
80. Paljor - Glorious
81. Dechen - Great Happiness
82. Chimi - Immortal
83. Namgyal - Victorious
84. Lobsang - Enlightened Mind
85. Karma - Action
86. Ngawang - Power of Speech
87. Rigzin - Knowledge Holder
88. Tsering - Long Life
89. Wangchuk - Mighty
90. Thubten - Buddha's Teachings
91. Yonten - Knowledgeable
92. Sangay - Buddha
93. Palden - Glorious
94. Kalden - Golden Age
95. Jamyang - Gentle Voice
96. Trinley - Buddha's Activities
97. Gyatso - Ocean
98. Sherab - Wisdom
99. Chogden - Supreme Dharma
100. Tseten - Firm Life

Maldivian baby names and their meanings

1. Aamaal - 'hope' or 'aspiration' in Maldivian
2. Aasiya - 'consoling' or 'comforting'
3. Afaaf - 'pure' or 'chaste'
4. Ahana - 'first ray of light'
5. Aisha - 'alive' or 'she who lives'
6. Ameen - 'trustworthy' or 'faithful'
7. Amjad - 'more glorious' or 'most noble'
8. Anaya - 'caring' or 'compassionate'
9. Asif - 'gather' or 'harvest'
10. Asiya - 'consoling' or 'nurturing'
11. Azhar - 'most shining' or 'luminous'
12. Badr - 'full moon'
13. Basim - 'smiling'
14. Bilal - 'water' or 'moistness'
15. Bushra - 'good news' or 'glad tidings'
16. Dalia - 'flower'
17. Dania - 'God is my judge'
18. Ehsan - 'perfection' or 'excellence'
19. Fadil - 'generous' or 'honorable'
20. Faisal - 'decisive' or 'resolute'
21. Farah - 'joy' or 'happiness'
22. Farid - 'unique' or 'matchless'
23. Fazal - 'grace' or 'favor'
24. Ghazal - 'love poem' or 'ode'
25. Gulzar - 'rose garden'
26. Hafsa - 'lioness'
27. Hani - 'happy' or 'content'
28. Hasan - 'handsome' or 'good'
29. Idris - 'interpreter'
30. Iman - 'faith' or 'belief'
31. Inaya - 'care' or 'protection'
32. Isra - 'nocturnal journey'
33. Javed - 'eternal' or 'everlasting'
34. Kamil - 'perfect' or 'complete'

35. Kareem - 'generous' or 'noble'
36. Khalid - 'eternal' or 'immortal'
37. Laila - 'night'
38. Latif - 'kind' or 'gentle'
39. Layla - 'night' or 'dark beauty'
40. Lubna - 'storax tree'
41. Mahir - 'skilled' or 'expert'
42. Mahmud - 'praiseworthy' or 'commendable'
43. Maimuna - 'blessed' or 'fortunate'
44. Majid - 'noble' or 'glorious'
45. Malika - 'queen'
46. Manal - 'achievement' or 'attainment'
47. Marjan - 'coral'
48. Masood - 'fortunate' or 'happy'
49. Munira - 'illuminating' or 'shining'
50. Nabeel - 'noble' or 'generous'
51. Nadia - 'the beginning' or 'first'
52. Nafisa - 'precious' or 'delicate'
53. Nahid - 'elevated' or 'generous'
54. Najeeb - 'noble' or 'of noble descent'
55. Naseem - 'breeze' or 'zephyr'
56. Nasir - 'helper' or 'supporter'
57. Nida - 'call' or 'voice'
58. Noor - 'light'
59. Qasim - 'one who distributes'
60. Rafiq - 'friend' or 'companion'
61. Rahim - 'merciful' or 'compassionate'
62. Rashid - 'rightly guided' or 'having true faith'
63. Rida - 'contentment' or 'satisfaction'
64. Sabah - 'morning'
65. Sadia - 'lucky' or 'fortunate'
66. Safa - 'purity' or 'clarity'
67. Salim - 'safe' or 'undamaged'
68. Sami - 'elevated' or 'sublime'
69. Samira - 'companion in evening conversation'
70. Shafiq - 'compassionate' or 'kind'

71. Shams - 'sun'
72. Sharif - 'noble' or 'honorable'
73. Suhail - 'canopus star'
74. Tahira - 'pure' or 'chaste'
75. Talib - 'seeker' or 'student'
76. Tamim - 'complete' or 'perfect'
77. Tariq - 'morning star'
78. Tasnim - 'a spring in paradise'
79. Umar - 'flourishing' or 'thriving'
80. Usman - 'baby bustard'
81. Wafa - 'faithfulness'
82. Yahya - 'God is gracious'
83. Yasir - 'wealthy'
84. Yousuf - 'God will increase'
85. Zafar - 'victory'
86. Zahir - 'bright' or 'shining'
87. Zahra - 'flower' or 'blossom'
88. Zain - 'beauty' or 'grace'
89. Zara - 'princess'
90. Zaynab - 'father's precious jewel'
91. Zeba - 'beautiful'
92. Ziad - 'growth' or 'increase'
93. Zohra - 'Venus' or 'beauty'
94. Zoya - 'alive' or 'life'
95. Zulaikha - 'brilliant beauty'
96. Zulfiqar - 'cleaver of the spine'
97. Zunaira - 'flower found in paradise'
98. Zahir - 'helper' or 'supporter'
99. Zaki - 'pure' or 'virtuous'
100. Zulaykha - 'beautiful'

Mauritian baby names and their meanings

1. Aashna - Hope and devotion
2. Abigail - Joy of the father
3. Aditi - Free and unbound
4. Aiden - Little fiery one
5. Akshay - Immortal, everlasting
6. Anaya - Caring, compassionate
7. Anushka - Grace, favor
8. Aria - Noble, melody
9. Arjun - Bright, shining
10. Arya - Noble, great
11. Avani - Earth
12. Bella - Beautiful, fair
13. Benjamin - Son of the right hand
14. Bhavna - Feelings, emotions
15. Chetan - Conscious, aware
16. Chloe - Blooming, fertility
17. Daniel - God is my judge
18. Darsh - Sight, vision
19. Devanshi - Divine
20. Dylan - Son of the sea
21. Eesha - Purity, desire
22. Emily - Industrious, striving
23. Ethan - Strong, firm
24. Freya - Noble woman, goddess of love
25. Gaurav - Pride, honor
26. Hannah - Grace, favor
27. Harsh - Happiness, joy
28. Isha - One who protects
29. Jack - God is gracious
30. Jai - Victory, triumph
31. Kaira - Peaceful, unique
32. Keshav - Another name of Lord Krishna
33. Kiara - Dark-haired, clear
34. Liam - Strong-willed warrior

35. Maanvi - Human, mankind
36. Mahi - The earth, great
37. Mia - Mine, beloved
38. Mohan - Charming, fascinating
39. Naina - Eyes, vision
40. Noah - Rest, comfort
41. Olivia - Olive tree, peace
42. Omkar - Sound of the sacred syllable Om
43. Pari - Angel, fairy
44. Pranav - Sacred syllable Om
45. Rhea - Flowing, river
46. Riya - Singer, graceful
47. Ryan - Little king
48. Saanvi - Goddess Lakshmi
49. Samaira - Enchanting, night talk
50. Tanvi - Beautiful, delicate
51. Uday - Rising, dawn
52. Vaibhav - Prosperity, wealth
53. Varun - Lord of the waters
54. Vedika - Consciousness, altar
55. William - Resolute protector
56. Xavier - Bright, splendid
57. Yash - Fame, glory
58. Zara - Blooming flower, princess
59. Aahana - Dawn, first light
60. Aarav - Peaceful, calm
61. Aanya - Grace, favor
62. Abhinav - New, young
63. Aditya - Sun, radiant
64. Aiden - Fiery one, strong
65. Anaya - Compassionate, caring
66. Aryan - Noble, spiritual
67. Ayush - Long life, age
68. Bella - Beautiful, fair
69. Benjamin - Son of the right hand
70. Chetan - Conscious, aware

71. Darsh - Sight, vision
72. Devanshi - Divine, heavenly
73. Emily - Hardworking, industrious
74. Ethan - Firm, enduring
75. Freya - Lady, noblewoman
76. Gaurav - Honor, pride
77. Hannah - Grace, favor
78. Isha - One who protects, night
79. Jack - God is gracious
80. Kaira - Peaceful, unique
81. Liam - Strong-willed warrior
82. Maanvi - Human, mankind
83. Mia - Mine, beloved
84. Noah - Rest, comfort
85. Olivia - Olive tree, peace
86. Pari - Fairy, angel
87. Riya - Singer, graceful
88. Ryan - Little king
89. Samaira - Enchanting, night talk
90. Tanvi - Beautiful, delicate
91. Uday - Rising, dawn
92. Vaibhav - Prosperity, wealth
93. William - Resolute protector
94. Xavier - Bright, splendid
95. Yash - Fame, glory
96. Zara - Princess, blooming flower
97. Aarush - First ray of the sun
98. Bhavya - Grand, splendid
99. Dhruv - Pole star, constant
100. Esha - Purity, desire

Seychellois baby names and their meanings

1. Aaron – High mountain
2. Abigail – Father's joy
3. Adeline – Noble
4. Adrian – Dark one
5. Agnes – Pure
6. Albert – Noble and bright
7. Alice – Noble
8. Alphonse – Ready for battle
9. Amelia – Industrious
10. Andre – Brave
11. Angela – Messenger of God
12. Anthony – Priceless
13. Aria – Air
14. Arthur – Bear
15. Ava – Bird
16. Benjamin – Son of the right hand
17. Bernadette – Brave as a bear
18. Bernard – Brave as a bear
19. Brigitte – Strength
20. Carl – Free man
21. Cecilia – Blind
22. Charles – Free man
23. Chloe – Green shoot
24. Christian – Follower of Christ
25. Claudia – Lame
26. Clement – Merciful
27. Daniel – God is my judge
28. David – Beloved
29. Denise – Follower of Dionysus
30. Diana – Divine
31. Dominic – Lord
32. Edith – Prosperous in war
33. Edward – Wealthy guardian
34. Elaine – Light

35. Elizabeth – God's promise
36. Emily – Industrious
37. Emma – Universal
38. Eric – Eternal ruler
39. Eugene – Well-born
40. Eva – Life
41. Felix – Happy
42. Florence – Flourishing
43. Francis – Free man
44. Gabriel – God is my strength
45. George – Farmer
46. Grace – Grace of God
47. Hannah – Grace of God
48. Harold – Army ruler
49. Helen – Bright
50. Henry – Ruler of the home
51. Isabella – Devoted to God
52. Jacob – Supplanter
53. James – Supplanter
54. Jean – God is gracious
55. Jessica – Rich
56. Joan – God is gracious
57. John – God is gracious
58. Joseph – God will increase
59. Julia – Youthful
60. Katherine – Pure
61. Kevin – Gentle
62. Laura – Laurel
63. Leo – Lion
64. Lisa – God's promise
65. Louis – Famous warrior
66. Lucy – Light
67. Margaret – Pearl
68. Maria – Bitter
69. Mark – Warlike
70. Martha – Lady

71. Martin – Warlike
72. Mary – Bitter
73. Matthew – Gift of God
74. Michael – Who is like God?
75. Monica – Advisor
76. Nancy – Grace
77. Natalie – Born on Christmas
78. Nicholas – Victory of the people
79. Nicole – Victory of the people
80. Olivia – Olive tree
81. Patrick – Noble
82. Paul – Small
83. Peter – Rock
84. Philip – Lover of horses
85. Rachel – Ewe
86. Rebecca – To tie
87. Richard – Brave ruler
88. Robert – Bright fame
89. Rose – Rose
90. Samuel – God has heard
91. Sarah – Princess
92. Simon – He has heard
93. Sophia – Wisdom
94. Stephen – Crown
95. Susan – Lily
96. Thomas – Twin
97. Victoria – Victory
98. Vincent – Conquering
99. William – Resolute protector
100. Zoe – Life

Malagasy baby names and their meanings

1. Aina - Life
2. Alain - Harmony
3. Andry - Warrior
4. Aro - Love
5. Bako - Blessing
6. Barijaona - Noble
7. Beri - Gift
8. Cid - Lord
9. Dera - Joy
10. Edmond - Wealthy protector
11. Faly - Happy
12. Fanja - Free
13. Fara - Beautiful
14. Feno - Fire
15. Gaby - God's strength
16. Haja - Respect
17. Iary - Light
18. Jaona - God is gracious
19. Kanto - Heart
20. Lala - Beloved
21. Lanto - Flame
22. Mamy - Sweet
23. Naly - Pure
24. Njaka - King
25. Ody - Journey
26. Parany - Brave
27. Rado - Loved one
28. Raja - King
29. Sitraka - Good luck
30. Tantely - Honey
31. Tojo - Wealth
32. Vola - Money
33. Zaka - Harvest
34. Zanahary - God

35. Adela - Noble
36. Bodo - Wisdom
37. Cela - Joyful
38. Dina - Judgement
39. Edwige - Fighter
40. Faneva - Eternal
41. Fifi - Jehovah increases
42. Gina - Queen
43. Hanta - Grace
44. Ilo - Sight
45. Joelle - God will add
46. Kanto - Heart
47. Lala - Beloved
48. Mampionona - Joyful
49. Nambina - Hope
50. Olivia - Olive tree
51. Patricia - Noble
52. Rahantamalala - Long-lasting happiness
53. Sabine - Woman of Sabine
54. Tiana - Princess
55. Veloma - Goodbye
56. Yasmine - Jasmine flower
57. Zara - Blooming flower
58. Ando - Light
59. Bemamy - Loved one
60. Christian - Follower of Christ
61. Dera - Joy
62. Elia - Jehovah is God
63. Faneva - Eternal
64. Gervais - Spear servant
65. Hery - Powerful ruler
66. Irina - Peace
67. Jaotombo - Great warrior
68. Kely - Little
69. Lanto - Flame
70. Mamy - Sweet

71. Naina - Eyes
72. Olivier - Olive tree
73. Parfait - Perfect
74. Rado - Loved one
75. Sitraka - Good luck
76. Tovo - Good
77. Voahangy - Angel
78. Zafy - Savior
79. Adela - Noble
80. Bina - Wisdom
81. Celina - Heaven
82. Doda - Beloved
83. Edwige - Fighter
84. Fara - Beautiful
85. Fifi - Jehovah increases
86. Gina - Queen
87. Hanta - Grace
88. Ilo - Sight
89. Joelle - God will add
90. Kanto - Heart
91. Lala - Beloved
92. Mampionona - Joyful
93. Nambina - Hope
94. Olivia - Olive tree
95. Patricia - Noble
96. Rahantamalala - Long-lasting happiness
97. Sabine - Woman of Sabine
98. Tiana - Princess
99. Veloma - Goodbye
100. Yasmine - Jasmine flower

Mauritanian baby names and their meanings

1. Aicha - alive
2. Ahmed - praised
3. Alia - exalted
4. Amadou - to praise God
5. Aminata - trustworthy
6. Bah - noble
7. Bintou - daughter of
8. Cheikh - elder
9. Cisse - master
10. Dede - mother
11. Djibril - God's strength
12. Ely - God's promise
13. Fatimata - captivating
14. Fode - replacement
15. Gueye - noble
16. Habib - beloved
17. Ibrahima - father of many
18. Ismail - God will hear
19. Jemal - beauty
20. Kadi - judge
21. Lamine - flourishing
22. Leila - night
23. Maimouna - blessed
24. Mariam - wished-for child
25. Mohamed - praiseworthy
26. Nana - grace
27. Oumar - long life
28. Penda - love
29. Rokia - health
30. Samba - second child
31. Tijani - crowned
32. Ummu - mother
33. Wane - God is gracious
34. Yacine - rich

35. Zeinab - fragrant flower
36. Abdoulaye - servant of God
37. Aissatou - woman of life
38. Babacar - father's friend
39. Coumba - with love
40. Djeneba - white
41. Elhadj - pilgrimage to Mecca
42. Fanta - beautiful day
43. Gorgui - master
44. Hawa - eve
45. Idrissa - immortal
46. Jamila - beautiful
47. Keba - born to bring joy
48. Lalla - lady
49. Mbacke - gift of God
50. Ndiaga - traveler
51. Ousmane - baby bustard
52. Ramata - golden
53. Sadio - pure
54. Talla - to ponder
55. Vieux - old
56. Yero - grandfather
57. Zalika - well-born
58. Adama - earth
59. Bamba - strong
60. Cheikhou - small elder
61. Daouda - beloved
62. Ebrima - father of multitude
63. Fatou - wean
64. Hadi - leader
65. Isse - God saves
66. Khadim - servant
67. Moustapha - chosen one
68. Ndeye - mother
69. Oumou - mother
70. Sidy - star

71. Talla - respected
72. Yakhya - God is gracious
73. Ablaye - God's servant
74. Boubacar - father's friend
75. Diarra - gift
76. Hamady - praiseworthy
77. Ibra - father of many
78. Khady - born premature
79. Mouhamed - praised one
80. Ndiouga - traveler
81. Seynabou - desert flower
82. Thierno - prince
83. Yande - mother
84. Aissata - woman of life
85. Binta - with God
86. Demba - one who endures
87. Hawa - longing
88. Issa - God is salvation
89. Kine - golden woman
90. Mame - mother
91. Ndeye - mother's love
92. Samba - second son
93. Thiam - lion
94. Yaye - mother
95. Amina - truthful
96. Bouna - prosperity
97. Diop - black
98. Hamet - praised
99. Idriss - studious
100. Kiné - queen

Gambian baby names and their meanings

1. Adama – Beautiful Child
2. Binta – Daughter
3. Cherno – Great
4. Dawda – Beloved
5. Ebrima – Father of the multitude
6. Fatou – Unique
7. Gibril – God is my strength
8. Hawa – Desired
9. Isatou – Love
10. Jatto – Strong
11. Kaddy – Pure
12. Lamin – Peace
13. Maimuna – Trustworthy
14. Njaga – Champion
15. Ousman – Powerful
16. Penda – Love
17. Quain – Intelligent
18. Rohey – Soul
19. Samba – Second boy
20. Tijan – Crown
21. Umi – Life
22. Vieux – Old
23. Wally – Loyal
24. Xale – Child
25. Yaya – Older brother
26. Zainab – Fragrant flower
27. Amie – Beloved
28. Baaba – Father's pride
29. Ceesay – Traveler
30. Demba – Peaceful
31. Ensa – Humanitarian
32. Foday – Born on a Friday
33. Gaoussou – Hidden treasure
34. Habib – Beloved

35. Ida – Hardworking
36. Jagne – Warrior
37. Kebba – Brave
38. Lala – Tulip
39. Mariama – Grace
40. Neneh – Mother
41. Oumie – Hope
42. Pa – Ocean
43. Quddus – Holy
44. Rama – Pleasing
45. Sainabou – Beautiful
46. Tamba – Brave
47. Umar – Long-lived
48. Vandi – Powerful
49. Wuyeh – Respected
50. Xolani – Peace
51. Yero – Gift from God
52. Zalika – Well-born
53. Awa – Beautiful angel
54. Bubacarr – Father's love
55. Coumba – Generous
56. Dodou – Beloved
57. Ebrima – Great one
58. Fatim – Captivating
59. Gano – Victory
60. Haddy – My delight
61. Ismaila – God will hear
62. Jaha – Dignity
63. Kumba – Joy
64. Lolley – Ruby
65. Mbye – Strong
66. Nana – Grace
67. Ousainou – Powerful
68. Pateh – Lion
69. Quamar – Moon
70. Ramatoulie – Bright star

71. Sainey – Beautiful
72. Tida – Sun
73. Uzoma – Good road
74. Vafing – Respectful
75. Wuri – Gold
76. Xola – Stay in peace
77. Yankuba – Honor
78. Zainaba – Beautiful flower
79. Ayisatou – Truthful
80. Baboucarr – Father's love
81. Cumba – Loved one
82. Duta – Eagle
83. Essa – God is salvation
84. Fama – Fame
85. Gassama – Kindness
86. Hagi – Pilgrimage
87. Idrissa – Immortal
88. Jallow – Peaceful
89. Kawsu – Pure
90. Lissa – Honey
91. Modou – Joy
92. Njogu – Elephant
93. Oumou – Hope
94. Pa Modou – Ocean's joy
95. Queenie – Queen
96. Rohey – Soul
97. Sise – Born on Sunday
98. Tapha – Crown
99. Uma – Nation
100. Yusef – God will increase

Senegalese baby names and their meanings

1. Aissatou - Peace
2. Abdou - Servant of God
3. Awa - Beautiful angel
4. Adama - Beautiful butterfly
5. Binta - Daughter
6. Babacar - Father's friend
7. Cheikh - Leader or chief
8. Coumba - One who is loved
9. Daouda - Beloved
10. Djibril - God is my strength
11. Fatou - Unique
12. Fode - Joy
13. Gora - Warrior
14. Hawa - Desired
15. Ibrahima - Father of many
16. Jallo - Light of the family
17. Kine - Golden
18. Lamine - Trustworthy
19. Mame - Born on a Saturday
20. Ndeye - Mother
21. Oumar - Long-lived
22. Penda - Loving one
23. Rokhaya - Star
24. Samba - Second son
25. Tidiane - Gift from God
26. Yacine - Rich in kindness
27. Zalika - Well-born
28. Ablaye - God's servant
29. Bineta - Daughter of satisfaction
30. Cisse - Ancient
31. Daba - Kind-hearted
32. Elhadji - One who has completed the Hajj
33. Fatima - Captivating
34. Gueye - Noble

35. Haby - Gift from God
36. Ismael - God will hear
37. Khadim - Servant
38. Lika - Angel
39. Moussa - Saved from the waters
40. Nafi - Beneficial
41. Ousmane - Young bird
42. Papa - Father
43. Rama - Pleasing
44. Seydou - Lucky
45. Talla - Knowledgeable
46. Yaye - Mother
47. Amina - Trustworthy
48. Boubacar - Great friend
49. Cheikhou - Little leader
50. Dior - Gold
51. Fallou - Respectful
52. Gorgui - Dignity
53. Hassana - Beautiful
54. Idrissa - Immortal
55. Keba - Earth
56. Matar - Rain
57. Ngor - Dignity
58. Oulimata - To stand out
59. Pape - Pope
60. Sadio - Pure
61. Thierno - Prince
62. Yoff - Seashore
63. Aissatou - Peaceful
64. Bouna - Beneficial
65. Cherif - Noble
66. Djeneba - White
67. Fatoumata - Daughter of the Prophet
68. Habib - Beloved
69. Imane - Faith
70. Khady - Born between two seasons

71. Lissa - Destiny
72. Ndeye - Mother
73. Ousseynou - Little wolf
74. Ramata - High, lofty
75. Sira - Journey
76. Tamsir - Guide
77. Yero - Father's love
78. Aicha - Living, prosperous
79. Badara - Full moon
80. Coumba - Loved one
81. Doudou - Beloved
82. Elhadj - Pilgrim
83. Fanta - Beautiful day
84. Gnilane - Graceful
85. Hamady - Praiseworthy
86. Isseu - Beautiful woman
87. Kader - Powerful
88. Mouhamed - Praised one
89. Ndiaga - Traveler
90. Oumy - Mother
91. Penda - Love
92. Saliou - Peaceful
93. Thiam - Lion
94. Yacouba - Supplanter
95. Amadou - To love God
96. Bocar - First born son
97. Cheikh - Leader
98. Diarra - Gift
99. Fadel - Excellent
100. Gueye - Respect

Guinean baby names and their meanings

1. Aissatou - the one who is loved
2. Almamy - It refers to a religious leader
3. Amara - grace or mercy
4. Binta - daughter
5. Camara - teacher
6. Dalanda - one who is admired
7. Diarra - gift
8. Fatoumata - the one who abstains
9. Hawa - desired or longed for
10. Ibrahima - father of many
11. Kadiatou - trustworthy
12. Lamine - knowledgeable
13. Mafoudia - the fortunate one
14. N'Fanly - handsome
15. Oumou - mother
16. Sadio - pure
17. Thierno - prince
18. Yarie - light
19. Zalikatou - blessed
20. Abdoulaye - servant of God
21. Aminata - trustworthy
22. Boubacar - father's friend
23. Coumba - the one who is loved
24. Djeneba - angel
25. Fanta - beautiful day
26. Hadja - pilgrimage
27. Ismael - God will hear
28. Karamoko - gift of God
29. Leila - night
30. Mamadou - praised one
31. Nene - girl
32. Oury - fire
33. Safiatou - pure
34. Tidiane - follower of Islam

35. Yacouba - follower
36. Zeinab - fragrant flower
37. Alfa - first
38. Awa - beautiful angel
39. Balla - strength
40. Cellou - messenger of God
41. Djenabou - blessed mother
42. Fode - he who is loved
43. Hadjara - one who migrates
44. Iye - mother
45. Keba - promise of God
46. Lounceny - God is gracious
47. Maimouna - blessed
48. N'Famara - loved one
49. Ousmane - baby bustard bird
50. Saliou - righteous
51. Tafsir - interpretation
52. Yaya - elder brother
53. Zainab - daughter of the prophet
54. Aly - exalted
55. Assiatou - one who is heard
56. Boubou - respected
57. Damba - dancer
58. Fadima - pure
59. Hassane - handsome
60. Idrissa - immortal
61. Kadija - premature child
62. Lansana - lion
63. Mariama - gift from God
64. N'Gady - happiness
65. Oumar - long-lived
66. Salim - peaceful
67. Tamba - rock
68. Yero - father's love
69. Zara - flower
70. Alhassane - good-looking

71. Assan - last
72. Bouba - great
73. Dian - light
74. Fanta - beautiful day
75. Hassimi - strong
76. Iye - mother
77. Kadi - pure
78. Lassana - handsome
79. Mariame - beloved
80. N'Golo - eagle
81. Ousseynou - little wolf
82. Salimatou - safe
83. Teli - angel
84. Yero - father's love
85. Zena - news
86. Alpha - first
87. Assiatou - one who is heard
88. Boubacar - father's friend
89. Djibril - God's promise
90. Fodeba - loved one
91. Hawa - desired
92. Ibrahima - father of many
93. Kante - love
94. Leno - joy
95. Momo - son
96. Naby - prophet
97. Oury - fire
98. Samba - second boy
99. Tidiani - follower of Islam
100. Yaguine - one who is loved

Ivorian baby names and their meanings

1. Abena - Born on Tuesday
2. Adjoa - Born on Monday
3. Ama - Born on Saturday
4. Akissi - Born after twins
5. Awa - Born on Thursday
6. Bamba - Born after twins
7. Binta - With God
8. Cisse - Ancient
9. Dabila - Born during a festival
10. Djeneba - Born after a great event
11. Ebere - Mercy
12. Fanta - Beautiful
13. Fode - Born after a great event
14. Gnamien - God's gift
15. Habiba - Beloved
16. Isha - Life
17. Jeneba - Born on Tuesday
18. Kablan - Born during harvest
19. Kadi - Pure
20. Lamine - Immortal
21. Maimouna - Blessed
22. Nana - Graceful
23. Ndeye - Mother
24. Oumou - Mother
25. Penda - Love
26. Quattara - Born during a journey
27. Rokia - Queen
28. Sira - Bright star
29. Teneba - Born during a journey
30. Umu - First born
31. Vamba - Born during a journey
32. Wassa - Born during a journey
33. Xalima - Peaceful
34. Yacouba - God will add

35. Zalika - Well born
36. Adama - Beautiful butterfly
37. Bintou - Daughter of joy
38. Coumba - Born on Friday
39. Djibril - God's strength
40. Esi - Born on Sunday
41. Fatou - Unique
42. Gnire - Born during harvest
43. Hadiya - Gift
44. Isata - Born on Monday
45. Jariatu - Born during a journey
46. Karamoko - Born after twins
47. Lala - Tulip
48. Mariam - Beloved
49. Nandi - Sweet
50. Oulimata - Born on Saturday
51. Penda - Loving
52. Quiana - Living with grace
53. Rougui - Born during a journey
54. Sana - Radiance
55. Tamba - Born after twins
56. Uma - Nation
57. Vafing - Born during a journey
58. Wassa - Born during a journey
59. Xolani - Peace
60. Yaa - Born on Thursday
61. Zainab - Fragrant flower
62. Adja - Born on Monday
63. Binti - Daughter
64. Coulibaly - Born on Friday
65. Djene - Born on Tuesday
66. Esso - Born on Sunday
67. Fatima - Captivating
68. Gnima - Born during harvest
69. Haby - Joyful
70. Issa - God is salvation

71. Jatta - Born during a journey
72. Kady - Pure
73. Laila - Night beauty
74. Marietou - Pure
75. Nafissatou - Precious
76. Oumy - Mother
77. Pemba - Born on Friday
78. Queen - Female monarch
79. Rama - Pleasing
80. Sadio - Born during a journey
81. Tia - Princess
82. Umaima - Little mother
83. Vafara - Born during a journey
84. Wassila - Born during a journey
85. Xena - Hospitable
86. Yafa - Beautiful
87. Zara - Blooming flower
88. Aicha - Living
89. Bineta - Daughter of satisfaction
90. Coumba - Born on Friday
91. Djibo - Born on Monday
92. Eunice - Victorious
93. Fatoumata - Daughter of the prophet
94. Gnagna - Born during harvest
95. Hawa - Desired
96. Ismael - God will hear
97. Jeneba - Born on Tuesday
98. Kadiatou - Pure
99. Lalla - Lady
100. Mariama - Pure

Burkinabe baby names and their meanings

1. Adama – Earth
2. Aissatou – The one who is cherished
3. Awa – Born on Friday
4. Bintou – Daughter of
5. Boureima – The first born after twins
6. Chantal – Song
7. Daouda – Beloved
8. Djeneba – The one who is beautiful
9. Elise – God is my oath
10. Fatoumata – The weaning
11. Fati – Captivating
12. Hama – Protector
13. Hassane – Handsome
14. Idrissa – Immortal
15. Issa – God is salvation
16. Kadiatou – The first born girl
17. Karim – Generous
18. Labiba – Wise
19. Madina – City of the Prophet
20. Mariam – Sea of bitterness
21. Moussa – Drawn out of the water
22. Nafissatou – Precious
23. Ousmane – Young snake
24. Patrice – Nobleman
25. Ramata – The high, exalted one
26. Salimata – Peaceful
27. Souleymane – Man of peace
28. Tidiane – Follower of the Tijaniyyah Sufi order
29. Yacouba – Supplanter
30. Zalissa – Successful
31. Zalika – Well-born
32. Zourata – The chosen one
33. Amina – Trustworthy
34. Bilal – Water

35. Cisse – Ancient
36. Djamila – Beautiful
37. Fatima – Captivating
38. Habib – Beloved
39. Ibrahima – Father of many
40. Kadi – Judge
41. Lamine – Flourishing
42. Moussa – Saved from the water
43. Naima – Comfort
44. Oumar – Long life
45. Rokia – Queen
46. Sadio – Lucky
47. Tahir – Pure
48. Yaya – Older brother
49. Zara – Flower
50. Zoumana – Protector
51. Abdoulaye – Servant of God
52. Binta – With God
53. Cheick – Leader
54. Djibril – God is my strength
55. Fanta – Beautiful day
56. Hamidou – Praiseworthy
57. Ismael – God will hear
58. Karamoko – Generous teacher
59. Latifa – Gentle
60. Maimouna – Blessed
61. Nana – Grace
62. Oumou – Mother
63. Rakia – Firmament
64. Sali – Righteous
65. Tene – Health
66. Yacine – Rich
67. Zahra – Flower
68. Zou – Sweet
69. Aicha – Living
70. Boubacar – Father of many

71. Coumba – The one who is loved
72. Djene – Mother
73. Fadimata – Unique
74. Halima – Gentle
75. Issouf – God will add
76. Kassim – Distributor
77. Leila – Night
78. Mamadou – Praised
79. Ndeye – Mother
80. Ousseynou – Little wolf
81. Ramatou – High
82. Salif – Predecessor
83. Thierno – Saint
84. Yero – The one who is loved
85. Zainab – Father's jewel
86. Zongo – Messenger
87. Ablavi – Life
88. Boubou – Dress
89. Daba – Goodness
90. Fifi – Jehovah increases
91. Hadi – Guide to righteousness
92. Isidore – Gift of Isis
93. Koffi – Born on Friday
94. Lassina – Protector
95. Marietou – Lady
96. N'da – Mother
97. Oumy – Mother
98. Rama – Pleasing
99. Samba – Second boy
100. Tidjane – Gift from God

Ghanaian baby names and their meanings

1. Aba – Born on Thursday
2. Adwoa – Born on Monday
3. Akosua – Born on Sunday
4. Afia – Born on Friday
5. Ama – Born on Saturday
6. Akua – Born on Wednesday
7. Abena – Born on Tuesday
8. Kofi – Born on Friday
9. Kwame – Born on Saturday
10. Kwabena – Born on Tuesday
11. Kwaku – Born on Wednesday
12. Yaw – Born on Thursday
13. Kojo – Born on Monday
14. Ekua – Born on Wednesday
15. Esi – Born on Sunday
16. Efua – Born on Friday
17. Kweku – Born on Wednesday
18. Kwesi – Born on Sunday
19. Akwetey – Born after twins
20. Akoto – First-born twin
21. Panyin – Elder twin
22. Kakra – Younger twin
23. Nana – Term of endearment, meaning King or Queen
24. Nyamekye – Gift from God
25. Adom – Grace
26. Akwasi – Born on Sunday
27. Amma – Born on Saturday
28. Kwadwo – Born on Monday
29. Obiara – Everyone's heart
30. Ohene – King
31. Ohemaa – Queen
32. Adjoa – Born on Monday
33. Adoma – Beautiful child

34. Afriyie – Born during good times
35. Akuafo – Farmer
36. Atoapem – Humility
37. Ayisi – Born on Sunday
38. Boatemaa – Born on Tuesday
39. Boakye – Born on Tuesday
40. Danso – Reliable
41. Ebo – Born on Tuesday
42. Ekow – Born on Thursday
43. Ewurabena – Born on Tuesday
44. Fiifi – Born on Friday
45. Gyamfi – Born on Friday
46. Kakra – Younger twin
47. Kesse – Born on Sunday
48. Kobby – Born on Tuesday
49. Kwamina – Born on Saturday
50. Kwasi – Born on Sunday
51. Maame – Mother
52. Nhyira – Blessing
53. Oforiwaa – Born on Tuesday
54. Oko – Born on Wednesday
55. Poku – Born on Wednesday
56. Tawiah – Born after a twin
57. Yaa – Born on Thursday
58. Yawson – Born on Thursday
59. Adusa – Thirteenth-born child
60. Afua – Born on Friday
61. Akoto – Second-born after twins
62. Ameyaw – Rejoicing in a son
63. Boahen – King's son
64. Dufie – Born on Friday
65. Kyei – Dignity
66. Mensah – Third-born son
67. Nsiah – Sixth-born child
68. Obeng – Born on Tuesday
69. Oheneba – Prince

70. Poku – Born on Wednesday
71. Serwaa – Noblewoman
72. Takyi – Respect
73. Yamoah – God's gift
74. Yaw – Born on Thursday
75. Adjei – Born on Monday
76. Adoma – Beautiful child
77. Afua – Born on Friday
78. Akua – Born on Wednesday
79. Amma – Born on Saturday
80. Boahen – King's son
81. Dufie – Born on Friday
82. Kyei – Dignity
83. Mensah – Third-born son
84. Nsiah – Sixth-born child
85. Obeng – Born on Tuesday
86. Oheneba – Prince
87. Poku – Born on Wednesday
88. Serwaa – Noblewoman
89. Takyi – Respect
90. Yamoah – God's gift
91. Yaw – Born on Thursday
92. Adjei – Born on Monday
93. Adoma – Beautiful child
94. Afua – Born on Friday
95. Akua – Born on Wednesday
96. Amma – Born on Saturday
97. Boahen – King's son
98. Dufie – Born on Friday
99. Kyei – Dignity
100. Mensah – Third-born son

Togolese baby names and their meanings

1. Abra - father of many nations
2. Adjoa - born on Monday
3. Afia - born on Friday
4. Afi - born on Friday
5. Akou - she who is loved
6. Akpene - thank you
7. Akua - born on Wednesday
8. Ami - my people
9. Aya - born on Friday
10. Ayawovi - we are rejoicing
11. Ayoko - born on Thursday
12. Dede - child of love
13. Dela - the savior
14. Dzifa - peaceful heart
15. Edem - God has saved me
16. Edna - rejuvenation
17. Ekoue - God's will
18. Ekua - born on Wednesday
19. Eli - God is great
20. Elom - God loves me
21. Enam - gift from God
22. Esi - born on Sunday
23. Esinam - God has heard me
24. Etornam - God has answered me
25. Eyram - God's grace
26. Fafa - peaceful
27. Fui - God's grace
28. Ganyo - money is good
29. Honam - God's gift
30. Kafui - praise Him
31. Kekeli - light
32. Koffi - born on Friday
33. Komla - death is inevitable
34. Kossi - born on Sunday

35. Kudjo - born on Monday
36. Kwabla - born on Tuesday
37. Kwame - born on Saturday
38. Kwasi - born on Sunday
39. Leena - light
40. Mawuena - God's doing
41. Mawuli - God exists
42. Mawuko - only God
43. Mawunyo - God is good
44. Mawusi - in the hands of God
45. Mawulolo - God is great
46. Mawuko - there is God
47. Naa - born on Thursday
48. Nana - king or queen
49. Nuku - great
50. Nyawo - mother's love
51. Ofori - sturdy tree
52. Povi - princess
53. Selasi - God heard me
54. Selorm - God loves me
55. Sika - money
56. Togbe - king
57. Yaa - born on Thursday
58. Yawa - born on Thursday
59. Yayra - blessing
60. Zanetor - darkness should cease
61. Zewuze - the world is sweet
62. Zikpui - promise
63. Zita - seeker
64. Ziwu - the universe
65. Zofia - wisdom
66. Zuna - happiness
67. Adzo - born on Monday
68. Abla - born on Wednesday
69. Afua - born on Friday
70. Akosua - born on Sunday

71. Ameyo - born on Saturday
72. Awo - born on Thursday
73. Dzidzor - joy
74. Elikplim - God is with me
75. Fiavi - princess
76. Kekeli - light
77. Klenam - leave it to God
78. Komla - death is inevitable
79. Kosi - born on Sunday
80. Mawulolo - God is great
81. Mawusi - in the hands of God
82. Nyawo - mother's love
83. Selorm - God loves me
84. Yayra - blessing
85. Zanetor - darkness should cease
86. Zewuze - the world is sweet
87. Zikpui - promise
88. Zita - seeker
89. Ziwu - the universe
90. Zofia - wisdom
91. Zuna - happiness
92. Adzo - born on Monday
93. Abla - born on Wednesday
94. Afua - born on Friday
95. Akosua - born on Sunday
96. Ameyo - born on Saturday
97. Awo - born on Thursday
98. Dzidzor - joy
99. Elikplim - God is with me
100. Fiavi - princess

Beninese baby names and their meanings

1. Abeni – We asked for her, and behold, we got her
2. Adeola – Crown of wealth
3. Afolabi – Born into high status
4. Akanni – Encounter brings possession
5. Alaba – Joy has come
6. Amara – Grace or mercy
7. Amina – Trustworthy and faithful
8. Ayotunde – Joy has returned
9. Babatunde – Father has returned
10. Bankole – Build my home for me
11. Chidinma – God is good
12. Chijioke – God is generous
13. Chima – God knows
14. Chinyere – God gave
15. Dada – Curly haired
16. Damisi – Cheerful
17. Dayo – Joy arrives
18. Ejiro – Praise God
19. Ekundayo – Sorrow becomes joy
20. Enitan – Person of story
21. Folami – Respect and honor me
22. Funmilayo – Give me joy
23. Gbenga – Lift up
24. Idowu – Born after twins
25. Ife – Love
26. Ige – Born feet first
27. Jumoke – Loved by everyone
28. Kehinde – The second-born of twins
29. Kola – Bring wealth
30. Morenike – I have someone to cherish
31. Ngozi – Blessing
32. Obi – Heart
33. Odion – First of twins
34. Ola – Wealth

35. Olanrewaju – My wealth is the future
36. Olufemi – God loves me
37. Olumide – My God has come
38. Omolara – A child is a comfort
39. Oni – Born on holy ground
40. Opeyemi – I give thanks
41. Osas – God's will
42. Sade – Honor confers a crown
43. Taiwo – Taste the world
44. Titi – Eternal
45. Toluwani – God's will
46. Uche – Thought
47. Yemi – Be fitting of me
48. Zuri – Beautiful
49. Olajumoke – Wealth meets with pampering
50. Adeyemi – The crown fits me
51. Bolanle – Finds wealth at home
52. Chisom – God is following me
53. Efe – Wealth
54. Femi – Love me
55. Ijeoma – Good journey
56. Kemi – Pamper me
57. Nkiru – The best is yet to come
58. Olabisi – Joy is multiplied
59. Oluwa – God
60. Simisola – Rest in wealth
61. Temitope – Enough to give thanks
62. Wale – Come home
63. Yewande – Mother has returned
64. Abioye – Born into royalty
65. Adetokunbo – The crown came from over the sea
66. Akin – Brave
67. Bukola – Add to the wealth
68. Chinedu – God leads
69. Ekaete – First daughter
70. Funke – Given to God to take care of

71. Ireti – Hope
72. Kola – Bring in wealth
73. Nkem – My own
74. Oladele – Wealth has come home
75. Olufunmilayo – God gives me joy
76. Oyin – Honey
77. Sola – Honor earns wealth
78. Temiloluwa – God's own
79. Wura – Gold
80. Yinka – Surrounding me with tenderness
81. Adisa – One who will teach us
82. Bolade – Honor arrives
83. Chika – God is supreme
84. Ekenedilichukwu – Thanks be to God
85. Foluke – Placed in God's hands
86. Iyabo – Mother has returned
87. Kosi – There's none like this
88. Nneka – Mother is supreme
89. Olajide – Wealth awakes
90. Olumuyiwa – God brought this
91. Oyindamola – Honey is mixed into wealth
92. Shola – Honor has entered
93. Tola – Wealth is the future
94. Wole – Enter the home
95. Yemi – Worth of me
96. Ademola – Crown is added to my wealth
97. Bolaji – Wake up in wealth
98. Chike – God's power
99. Ekenwa – Wealth is a child
100. Folade – Honor brings wealth

Nigerian baby names and their meanings

1. Adeola – Crown of wealth
2. Adesuwa – One who brings joy
3. Afolabi – Born into high status
4. Akachi – Hand of God
5. Akinyemi – Fated to be a warrior
6. Amaka – Precious child
7. Amina – Peaceful, safe
8. Ayodele – Joy comes home
9. Babatunde – Father has returned
10. Bolade – Honor arrives
11. Chidiebere – God is merciful
12. Chidubem – God is my guide
13. Chijioke – God holds a share
14. Chike – God's power
15. Chima – God knows
16. Chinedu – God leads
17. Chisom – God follows me
18. Daberechi – Lean on God
19. Damilola – God makes me wealthy
20. Efe – Wealth
21. Ekenedilichukwu – Thanks be to God
22. Emeka – Great deeds
23. Eniola – Person of wealth
24. Enitan – Person of story
25. Esosa – God's gift
26. Femi – Love me
27. Folami – Honor me
28. Funmilayo – Give me joy
29. Gbemisola – Carry me into wealth
30. Habiba – Beloved
31. Halima – Gentle, patient
32. Idowu – Born after twins
33. Ifeoluwa – Love of God
34. Ifunanya – Love inspires love

35. Ige – Born feet-first
36. Ikechukwu – Power of God
37. Isioma – Good luck
38. Jadesola – Come into wealth
39. Kehinde – Second-born of twins
40. Kola – Bring wealth
41. Morenike – I have someone to cherish
42. Ngozi – Blessing
43. Njideka – I have what is greater
44. Nkem – My own
45. Nkemdilim – My own is mine
46. Obi – Heart
47. Olabisi – Joy is multiplied
48. Olamide – My wealth has come
49. Olufemi – God loves me
50. Olumide – God has arrived
51. Onyeka – Who is greater than God
52. Opeyemi – I give thanks
53. Oreoluwa – Gift of God
54. Oyin – Honey
55. Rotimi – Stay with me
56. Sade – Honor confers a crown
57. Simisola – Rest in wealth
58. Taiwo – Taste the world
59. Temiloluwa – God's own
60. Toluwalope – God's will
61. Uchechi – God's will
62. Uzoma – Good way
63. Wuraola – Gold of wealth
64. Yewande – Mother has returned
65. Zainab – Father's jewel
66. Abidemi – Born during father's absence
67. Adanna – Her father's daughter
68. Ademola – Crown brings happiness
69. Aderonke – Crown has something to pamper
70. Ajani – He fights for possession

71. Akanni – Encounter brings possession
72. Anwuli – Joy is great
73. Azuka – Back is greater
74. Bankole – Build my home
75. Bolanle – Find wealth at home
76. Bukola – Add to the wealth
77. Chibuike – God is strength
78. Chidinma – God is good
79. Chinyere – God gives
80. Durosinmi – Wait to rest
81. Ebunoluwa – Gift from God
82. Enitan – Story personified
83. Folasade – Use wealth as a crown
84. Ireti – Hope
85. Jumoke – Everyone loves the child
86. Kikelomo – Child to be pampered
87. Modupe – I am grateful
88. Moradeke – I have found something to pamper
89. Nkiru – The best is yet to come
90. Olajumoke – Wealth meets a child
91. Olufunmilayo – God gives me joy
92. Oluwakemi – God pampers me
93. Oluwatoyin – God is worthy to be praised
94. Omolara – A child is a benefit
95. Onome – My own
96. Temidayo – My life has turned to joy
97. Titilayo – Everlasting joy
98. Yemisi – Honor me
99. Yetunde – Mother has returned
100. Zikora – Show the world

Cameroonian baby names and their meanings

1. Abena - Born on Tuesday
2. Adamma - Beautiful girl
3. Ama - Born on Saturday
4. Akono - Firstborn
5. Akua - Born on Wednesday
6. Ayo - Joy
7. Binta - With God
8. Chidi - God exists
9. Chika - God is supreme
10. Chinyere - God's gift
11. Dada - Curly hair
12. Ebele - Mercy, kindness
13. Efia - Born on Friday
14. Ekaette - First daughter
15. Ekon - Strong
16. Eniola - Wealthy person
17. Eshe - Life
18. Femi - Love me
19. Folami - Respect and honor me
20. Gwandoya - Met with joy
21. Ife - Love
22. Isi - Born on Sunday
23. Jengo - Building
24. Kande - Firstborn daughter
25. Kato - Second of twins
26. Kehinde - Last born
27. Kesi - Born when the father had troubles
28. Kunto - Third born
29. Lekan - My wealth is increasing
30. Madu - People
31. Makena - The happy one
32. Makena - The happy one
33. Nia - Purpose

34. Ngozi - Blessing
35. Nia - Purpose
36. Nkiru - Good is the best
37. Obi - Heart
38. Ola - Wealth
39. Oni - Born on holy ground
40. Onyeka - Who is greater than God
41. Ozioma - Good news
42. Pili - Second born
43. Sade - Honor confers a crown
44. Taiwo - Taste the world
45. Tola - Wealth is the future
46. Uche - Thought
47. Udu - Clay pot
48. Ugo - Eagle
49. Ukeme - Ability
50. Uzoma - Good way
51. Yewande - Mother came back
52. Zola - Quiet, tranquil
53. Zuri - Beautiful
54. Adaeze - King's daughter
55. Akachi - Hand of God
56. Amara - Grace
57. Chiamaka - God is beautiful
58. Chijindu - God holds life
59. Chizoba - God save us
60. Ebelechukwu - Mercy of God
61. Ifeoma - Good thing
62. Ijeoma - Good journey
63. Nkechi - God's own
64. Nkemdilim - My own is in God's hand
65. Obiageli - One who has come to enjoy
66. Oluchi - God's work
67. Onyinyechi - Gift from God
68. Uchechi - God's will
69. Urenna - Father's pride

70. Zikora - Show the world
71. Adegoke - The crown has been exalted
72. Akintoye - Valor is worth joy
73. Babatunde - Father has returned
74. Chukwuma - God knows
75. Ekenedilichukwu - Thanks be to God
76. Ifeanyichukwu - Nothing is impossible with God
77. Ikenna - Power of God
78. Kelechi - Praise God
79. Nnamdi - My father is alive
80. Obinna - Father's heart
81. Olumide - My God has arrived
82. Onyekachi - Who is greater than God
83. Uchenna - God's thought
84. Ugochukwu - Glory of God
85. Chibuzo - God leads
86. Chinedu - God guides
87. Chukwudi - God exists
88. Emeka - Great deeds
89. Ikechukwu - Power of God
90. Nkem - My own
91. Okechukwu - God's portion
92. Onochie - One who replaces
93. Uzochi - God's way
94. Chijioke - God is the provider
95. Chukwuebuka - God is big
96. Eze - King
97. Ifeanyi - Nothing is impossible
98. Iheanacho - What we are looking for
99. Nnamdi - My father lives
100. Udo - Peace

Gabonese baby names and their meanings

1. Abame – one who is loved
2. Abena – born on Tuesday
3. Adamma – beautiful girl
4. Adanne – her mother's daughter
5. Adelaja – crown has honor
6. Afolabi – born into high status
7. Akachi – the hand of God
8. Akosua – born on Sunday
9. Akwete – older of twins
10. Alaba – joy has arrived
11. Ama – born on Saturday
12. Amara – grace
13. Anuli – joyful
14. Anyim – my own
15. Ayo – joy
16. Azuka – support is greater
17. Bem – peace
18. Chi – God
19. Chiamaka – God is beautiful
20. Chidi – God is there
21. Chijioke – God holds share
22. Chika – God is supreme
23. Chima – God knows
24. Chinelo – God thinks for me
25. Chinedu – God leads
26. Chinyere – God gives
27. Chisom – God follows me
28. Daberechi – lean on God
29. Dike – hero
30. Dumaka – help me praise God
31. Ebele – mercy, kindness
32. Echi – tomorrow
33. Ejiro – praise God
34. Ekene – praise

35. Emeka – great deeds
36. Eze – king
37. Femi – love me
38. Gbenga – lift up
39. Ife – love
40. Ifeanyi – nothing is impossible with God
41. Ifechi – light of God
42. Ifedayo – love brings happiness
43. Ifekristi – light of Christ
44. Ijeoma – safe journey
45. Ikechukwu – power of God
46. Ikenwa – child is more than money
47. Ireti – hope
48. Isioma – good luck
49. Jide – hold on
50. Kachi – God's will
51. Kainyechukwuekene – let's praise God
52. Kanu – eagle
53. Kelechi – praise God
54. Kenechukwu – thank God
55. Kosi – there's none
56. Kwame – born on Saturday
57. Lekan – my wealth is increasing
58. Lotanna – remember God
59. Mfon – grace
60. Ngozi – blessing
61. Nkem – my own
62. Nkemdilim – let mine be mine
63. Nkiru – the best is yet to come
64. Nkoli – remember parents
65. Nnamdi – my father is alive
66. Nneka – mother is supreme
67. Nwabueze – child is king
68. Nwanneka – siblings are supreme
69. Obi – heart
70. Obioma – kind heart

71. Ogechi – God's time
72. Okeke – born on Eke (market day)
73. Okoro – man
74. Okoye – born on Oye (farming day)
75. Oluchi – God's work
76. Onyeka – who is greater than God
77. Onyekachi – who is greater than God
78. Ozioma – good news
79. Somtochukwu – praise God with me
80. Uche – will
81. Uchechi – God's will
82. Uchenna – God's will
83. Ugo – eagle
84. Ugochi – God's pride
85. Uzoma – good way
86. Zikora – show the world
87. Zikoranachidimma – show the world that my God is good
88. Zina – God's gift
89. Ada – first daughter
90. Adaeze – king's daughter
91. Adaku – daughter born into wealth
92. Adanna – father's daughter
93. Adanne – her mother's daughter
94. Chioma – good God
95. Chinyere – God's gift
96. Ebere – mercy
97. Ijeoma – good journey
98. Ngozi – blessing
99. Nneka – mother is supreme
100. Uzoamaka – good journey

Equatorial Guinean baby names and their meanings

1. Abayomi - brings joy in Fang
2. Adaeze - king's daughter in Bubi
3. Afamefuna - my name will not be lost in Fang
4. Akachi - the hand of God in Bubi
5. Akuchi - wealth from God in Fang
6. Amara - grace in Bubi
7. Amaugo - sweet life in Fang
8. Anuli - joy in Bubi
9. Azubuike - back is strength in Fang
10. Chiamaka - God is beautiful in Bubi
11. Chibuzo - God leads the way in Fang
12. Chidera - once God has written in Bubi
13. Chidiebere - God is merciful in Fang
14. Chidimma - God is good in Bubi
15. Chijioke - God holds share in Fang
16. Chika - God is the greatest in Bubi
17. Chike - God's power in Fang
18. Chikere - God created in Bubi
19. Chinasa - God answers in Fang
20. Chinelo - God thinks for me in Bubi
21. Chinedu - God leads in Fang
22. Chinwe - God owns in Bubi
23. Chinyere - God gives in Fang
24. Chizoba - God protect us in Bubi
25. Chukwuma - God knows in Fang
26. Ebere - mercy in Bubi
27. Echezona - do not forget God in Fang
28. Echidime - God says in Bubi
29. Ejiro - praise God in Fang
30. Ekene - praise in Bubi
31. Emeka - great deeds in Fang
32. Emenike - God does things in Bubi
33. Enyinnaya - his father's friend in Fang

34. Ezinne - good mother in Bubi
35. Ifeanyi - nothing is impossible with God in Fang
36. Ifeoma - good thing in Bubi
37. Ifunanya - love in Fang
38. Iheanacho - what we are looking for in Bubi
39. Ijeoma - good journey in Fang
40. Ikenna - father's power in Bubi
41. Ijeawele - safe journey in Fang
42. Ikenwa - child of strength in Bubi
43. Kelechi - praise God in Fang
44. Kosisochukwu - as it pleases God in Bubi
45. Lotachi - remember God in Fang
46. Makuachukwu - embrace God in Bubi
47. Nchedochukwu - God's protection in Fang
48. Ngozi - blessing in Bubi
49. Njideka - one who is cherished in Fang
50. Nkechi - God's own in Bubi
51. Nkem - my own in Fang
52. Nkemdilim - let mine be in Bubi
53. Nkeiruka - the best is yet to come in Fang
54. Nkiru - the best is ahead in Bubi
55. Nnenna - father's mother in Fang
56. Nneoma - good mother in Bubi
57. Nwabueze - child is king in Fang
58. Nwanneka - siblings are supreme in Bubi
59. Nwanyibuife - a woman is light in Fang
60. Obi - heart in Bubi
61. Obioma - kind hearted in Fang
62. Obinna - father's heart in Bubi
63. Ogechi - God's time in Fang
64. Okechukwu - God's portion in Bubi
65. Okwukwe - faith in Fang
66. Oluchi - God's work in Bubi
67. Onyeka - who is superior to God in Fang
68. Onyekachi - who is greater than God in Bubi
69. Onyinye - gift in Fang

70. Ozioma -   good news in Bubi
71. Somtochukwu -   follow me to praise God in Fang
72. Uchenna -   God's will in Bubi
73. Ugochukwu -   God's pride in Fang
74. Ukamaka -   hard to know in Bubi
75. Uzochi -   God's way in Fang
76. Uzoma -   good path in Bubi
77. Zikora -   show the world in Fang
78. Zimuzo -   show me the way in Bubi
79. Ada -   first daughter in Fang
80. Adaku -   daughter born into wealth in Bubi
81. Adamma -   beautiful daughter in Fang
82. Akudo -   peaceful wealth in Bubi
83. Akuabia -   wealth has come in Fang
84. Akubundu -   wealth is life in Bubi
85. Akudinobi -   wealth is in the heart in Fang
86. Akunna -   father's wealth in Bubi
87. Amaka -   beautiful in Fang
88. Amakulor -   beauty of life in Bubi
89. Amaogechukwu -   God's time is the best in Fang
90. Chiamaka -   God is great in Bubi
91. Chidimma -   God is good in Fang
92. Chidozie -   God fixes it in Bubi
93. Chika -   God is supreme in Fang
94. Chinyere -   God gave in Bubi
95. Ebele -   mercy, kindness in Fang
96. Ifeoma -   a good thing in Bubi
97. Ijeoma -   good journey in Fang
98. Ngozi -   blessing in Bubi
99. Nkechi -   God's own in Fang
100. Uchechi -   God's will in Bubi

Congolese baby names and their meanings

1. Abeni – Prayed for
2. Abiba – Child born after grandmother died
3. Adaeze – Princess
4. Adanna – Father's daughter
5. Adanne – Mother's daughter
6. Adeola – Crown of wealth
7. Adisa – One who will teach us
8. Adjoa – Born on Monday
9. Afolabi – Born into high status
10. Afua – Born on Friday
11. Akachi – Hand of God
12. Akosua – Born on Sunday
13. Akua – Born on Wednesday
14. Ama – Born on Saturday
15. Amaka – Goodness, beauty
16. Amara – Grace
17. Amare – Handsome
18. Amina – Trustworthy, faithful
19. Ayo – Joy
20. Azibo – Earth
21. Binta – With God
22. Bolaji – Wake up in wealth
23. Chika – God is supreme
24. Chima – God knows
25. Chinara – God receives
26. Chinelo – God thinks for me
27. Chinue – God's blessing
28. Chinyere – God gave
29. Chisom – God follows me
30. Dabir – Teacher
31. Dada – Curly hair
32. Dalili – Sign
33. Deka – All will be well
34. Ebele – Mercy, kindness

35. Efe – Wealth
36. Efia – Born on Friday
37. Ekon – Strong
38. Eshe – Life
39. Femi – Love me
40. Folami – Honor me
41. Gamba – Warrior
42. Hasani – Handsome
43. Ife – Love
44. Ifeoma – Good thing
45. Ifunanya – Love inspires love
46. Ige – Born by breech
47. Imani – Faith
48. Isabis – Something beautiful
49. Isi – Born on Sunday
50. Jengo – Building
51. Jengo – One with a strong building
52. Kamaria – Like the moon
53. Kande – Firstborn daughter
54. Kato – Second of twins
55. Keji – Second born
56. Kesi – Born when father was in trouble
57. Kibibi – Little lady
58. Kofi – Born on Friday
59. Kojo – Born on Monday
60. Kwame – Born on Saturday
61. Kwasi – Born on Sunday
62. Lekan – My wealth is increasing
63. Leti – Joy
64. Makena – The happy one
65. Makena – Happy one
66. Malaika – Angel
67. Mandisa – Sweet
68. Masozi – Tears
69. Mbali – Flower
70. Mchumba – Sweetheart

71. Mirembe – Peace
72. Mosi – Firstborn
73. Nia – Purpose
74. Nia – Purpose, goal
75. Nkechi – God's own
76. Nneka – Mother is supreme
77. Ngozi – Blessing
78. Nia – Purpose
79. Nneka – Mother is supreme
80. Nsia – Sixth born child
81. Nuru – Light
82. Obi – Heart
83. Olabisi – Joy is multiplying
84. Olufemi – God loves me
85. Omari – God the highest
86. Oni – Born on holy ground
87. Onyeka – Who is greater than God
88. Rashidi – Thinker
89. Sade – Honor confers a crown
90. Sefu – Sword
91. Tandie – Fire
92. Tau – Lion
93. Thabo – Happiness
94. Uchechi – God's will
95. Uchenna – God's thoughts
96. Ugochi – Eagle of God
97. Uzoma – Good way
98. Winda – Hunting
99. Zola – Quiet, tranquil
100. Zuri – Beautiful

Angolan baby names and their meanings

1. Adao -   Son of the Red Earth
2. Adelia -   Noble Kind
3. Adelino -   Noble
4. Adelmo -   Noble Protector
5. Adriano -   From Hadria
6. Agostinho -   The Exalted One
7. Albano -   From Alba
8. Alda -   Old
9. Aleixo -   Defender
10. Aloisio -   Famous Warrior
11. Amalia -   Work
12. Amaro -   Dark
13. Ana -   Grace
14. Anabela -   Graceful Beauty
15. Anacleto -   Invoked
16. Anastacio -   Resurrection
17. Andre -   Manly
18. Angela -   Messenger of God
19. Anibal -   Grace of Baal
20. Antonia -   Priceless
21. Antonio -   Priceless
22. Armando -   Soldier
23. Artur -   Bear
24. Balbina -   Stammerer
25. Benvinda -   Welcome
26. Bernardo -   Strong as a Bear
27. Branca -   White
28. Bruno -   Brown
29. Caetano -   From Gaeta
30. Camila -   Young Ceremonial Attendant
31. Carlito -   Free Man
32. Carlos -   Free Man
33. Cecilia -   Blind
34. Celestino -   Heavenly

35. Cesar - Long Haired
36. Clara - Bright, Clear
37. Claudio - Lame
38. Clemente - Merciful
39. Conceicao - Conception
40. Corina - Maiden
41. Cristovao - Bearer of Christ
42. Damiao - To Tame
43. Daniel - God is My Judge
44. Dario - Possess
45. David - Beloved
46. Diana - Divine
47. Dina - Judged
48. Diogo - Doctrine
49. Domingos - Belonging to the Lord
50. Duarte - Wealthy Guardian
51. Dulce - Sweet
52. Edite - Prosperous in War
53. Eduardo - Wealthy Guardian
54. Elias - The Lord is My God
55. Elma - Will, Desire
56. Elsa - God's Promise
57. Emilio - Rival
58. Ermelinda - Universal Woman
59. Ernesto - Serious
60. Estevao - Crown
61. Eugenio - Well Born
62. Fabio - Bean Grower
63. Fatima - Captivating
64. Felipe - Friend of Horses
65. Fernanda - Adventurous
66. Fernando - Adventurous
67. Filomena - Friend of Strength
68. Flavio - Yellow Hair
69. Francisco - Free Man
70. Gabriel - God is My Strength

71. Gaspar - Treasurer
72. Geraldo - Ruler with a Spear
73. Gertrudes - Strength of a Spear
74. Gilberto - Bright Pledge
75. Graca - Grace
76. Gregorio - Vigilant, Watchful
77. Guilherme - Resolute Protector
78. Gustavo - Staff of the Goths
79. Helena - Light
80. Henrique - Home Ruler
81. Hermenegildo - Sacrifice
82. Hilda - Battle Woman
83. Hugo - Mind, Intellect
84. Humberto - Bright Support
85. Ines - Pure
86. Irene - Peace
87. Isabela - God is My Oath
88. Isidoro - Gift of Isis
89. Jacinta - Hyacinth
90. Joao - God is Gracious
91. Joaquim - Established by God
92. Jorge - Farmer
93. Jose - He Will Add
94. Juliana - Youthful
95. Julio - Youthful
96. Justino - Just, Fair
97. Laura - Laurel
98. Leandro - Lion Man
99. Leonor - Light
100. Leticia - Joy, Happiness

Namibian baby names and their meanings

1. Aina - forever
2. Amara - grace
3. Buhle - beauty
4. Chipo - gift
5. Dumi - inspiration
6. Esi - Sunday
7. Femi - love me
8. Gugu - precious
9. Hlengiwe - redeemed
10. Ina - pure
11. Jengo - building
12. Kaya - home
13. Lebo - thankful
14. Mudiwa - beloved
15. Nia - purpose
16. Oba - ruler
17. Pendo - love
18. Qhawe - hero
19. Rudo - love
20. Sipho - gift
21. Tandi - love
22. Udo - peace
23. Vuyo - joy
24. Wanga - possess
25. Xola - stay in peace
26. Yara - butterfly
27. Zola - quiet
28. Afua - born on Friday
29. Bako - first-born
30. Chuma - wealth
31. Dada - curly hair
32. Ebo - born on Tuesday
33. Fola - honor
34. Goma - drum

35. Hadiya - gift
36. Imani - faith
37. Jabu - joy
38. Kali - energetic
39. Langa - sun
40. Malaika - angel
41. Nandi - sweet
42. Oba - king
43. Paka - cat
44. Qalbi - my heart
45. Retha - excellent
46. Sanaa - work of art
47. Tawana - we have been loved
48. Uzuri - beauty
49. Vida - life
50. Wambui - singer of songs
51. Xhosa - sweet
52. Yemi - worthy of respect
53. Zuri - beautiful
54. Ayo - joy
55. Bonga - gratitude
56. Chidori - bird of luck
57. Deka - pleasing
58. Eshe - life
59. Fadhili - kindness
60. Gamba - warrior
61. Haki - justice
62. Ige - born by breech
63. Jengo - one who builds
64. Kito - precious child
65. Lulu - pearl
66. Mandisa - sweet
67. Nia - purpose
68. Oba - king
69. Pili - second
70. Qwara - divide

71. Raha - happiness
72. Siti - lady
73. Tendai - thankful
74. Uzima - vitality
75. Vita - war
76. Wendo - love
77. Xola - stay in peace
78. Yaa - born on Thursday
79. Zawadi - gift
80. Aisha - life
81. Buhle - beauty
82. Chuma - treasure
83. Dalili - sign
84. Eshe - life
85. Femi - love me
86. Gugu - precious
87. Hadiya - gift
88. Ife - love
89. Jabari - brave
90. Kali - energetic
91. Lulu - pearl
92. Mandla - strength
93. Nia - purpose
94. Oba - king
95. Penda - love
96. Qwara - divide
97. Rudo - love
98. Sana - brightness
99. Tendai - thankful
100. Uzuri - beauty

Botswanan baby names and their meanings

1. Abena - Born on a Tuesday
2. Adamma - Beautiful girl
3. Afia - Born on a Friday
4. Akua - Born on a Wednesday
5. Amara - Grace or kindness
6. Anaya - Look up to God
7. Ayo - Joy
8. Bontle - Beauty
9. Chipo - Gift
10. Dikeledi - Tears
11. Eshe - Life
12. Fola - Honor
13. Gontse - It is God's will
14. Hlengiwe - Rescued
15. Itumeleng - Joy
16. Jabulani - Rejoice
17. Kago - My little one
18. Katlego - Success
19. Lerato - Love
20. Lindiwe - Have waited
21. Masego - Blessings
22. Naledi - Star
23. Neo - Gift
24. Obakeng - Worship
25. Palesa - Flower
26. Rethabile - We are happy
27. Sefako - Praise
28. Thabo - Happiness
29. Tsholofelo - Hope
30. Uyapo - He will add
31. Zuri - Beautiful
32. Amogelang - Receive
33. Bame - Mother of kings
34. Bonolo - Ease

35. Ditshego - Laughter
36. Goitsemodimo - God knows
37. Karabo - Answer
38. Keitumetse - I am happy
39. Lesedi - Light
40. Mpho - Gift
41. Ontibile - He is with me
42. Rebaone - We are thankful
43. Segomotso - Comfort
44. Tshenolo - Wisdom
45. Thato - Will or desire
46. Boitumelo - Joy
47. Gaone - It is mine
48. Kagiso - Peace
49. Lebogang - Be thankful
50. Moagi - Builder
51. Neo - Gift
52. Oarabile - He loves us
53. Refilwe - We were given
54. Tebogo - Thanks
55. Tumisang - Praise
56. Othusitse - He has helped
57. Botshelo - Life
58. Goitseone - God knows
59. Keabetswe - We are given
60. Lethabo - Joy
61. Mphoentle - Beautiful gift
62. Omphile - He gave me
63. Rorisang - Praise
64. Seipati - Trust
65. Tuelo - Payment
66. Tumelo - Faith
67. Ofentse - He has conquered
68. Bokamoso - Future
69. Gape - Moreover
70. Kealeboga - I am thankful

71. Lorato - Love
72. Motheo - Foundation
73. Nthabiseng - Make me happy
74. Odirile - He is still alive
75. Reitumetse - We are pleased
76. Setshwano - Culture
77. Tshepiso - Promise
78. Tumisang - Praise
79. Onneile - He has given me
80. Bophelo - Life
81. Gofaone - He forgave me
82. Keamogetse - I have received
83. Letlhogonolo - Fortune
84. Moitshepi - Believer
85. Nthabeleng - Make me happy
86. Oagile - He has paid
87. Relebogile - We are thankful
88. Sontaga - Sunday
89. Tshepo - Trust
90. Tumelo - Faith
91. Oaitse - He knows me
92. Boitshoko - Perseverance
93. Goitsemang - Who knows?
94. Kelebogile - I am thankful
95. Letlotlo - Treasure
96. Moagi - Builder
97. Nthabiseng - Make me happy
98. Oabile - He has opened
99. Realeboga - We are thankful
100. Sefora - Bird

Zimbabwean baby names and their meanings

1. Tadiwa – We have been loved
2. Tafadzwa – We are pleased
3. Tafara – We are happy
4. Takudzwa – We have been honored
5. Tanaka – We are good
6. Tatenda – We are thankful
7. Tawanda – We are multiplied
8. Tendai – Be thankful
9. Tinashe – God is with us
10. Tsitsi – Mercy
11. Vimbai – Trust
12. Zivai – Know yourself
13. Anashe – With God
14. Anotida – We love him/her
15. Anotidaishe – We love him/her a lot
16. Ruvimbo – Hope
17. Rudo – Love
18. Shungu – Desire
19. Shupikai – Be quiet
20. Simbarashe – Power of the Lord
21. Tapiwa – Given
22. Tatenda – Grateful
23. Tavonga – With thanks
24. Tawana – We have
25. Tawonga – We are thankful
26. Thandiwe – Beloved
27. Tonderai – Look at
28. Tsungi – Praise
29. Vongai – Humility
30. Munashe – With God
31. Mufaro – Joy
32. Kundai – Love one another
33. Kuziva – Knowing

34. Mudiwa – Beloved
35. Natsai – Be agreeable
36. Nyasha – Grace
37. Panashe – With God
38. Rufaro – Happiness
39. Shingai – Be brave
40. Takunda – We have won
41. Tariro – Hope
42. Tendekai – Be willing
43. Tinotenda – We thank you
44. Tonderai – Consider
45. Vongai – Be humble
46. Zvikomborero – Blessing
47. Chenai – Cleanse
48. Chido – Desire
49. Farai – Be happy
50. Gamuchirai – Be open
51. Kudzai – Praise
52. Munyaradzi – Comforter
53. Ngoni – Of the Ngoni tribe
54. Nyarai – Be humble
55. Paidamoyo – For what the heart holds
56. Ruvarashe – Flower of the Lord
57. Shungudzo – Thought
58. Tadiwanashe – Loved by God
59. Tanyaradzwa – We have been comforted
60. Tashinga – We are strong
61. Tendai – Be thankful
62. Tinashe – God is with us
63. Tsungirirai – Be patient
64. Tapiwanashe – Given by God
65. Chiedza – Light
66. Dzidzai – Learn
67. Farirai – Look at
68. Gamuchirai – Be open
69. Kudakwashe – Will of God

70. Mufaro – Joy
71. Ngonidzashe – God's presence
72. Nyasha – Grace
73. Panashe – With God
74. Rufaro – Happiness
75. Shingirai – Look at
76. Takunda – We have won
77. Tariro – Hope
78. Tendekai – Be willing
79. Tinotenda – We thank you
80. Tonderai – Consider
81. Vongai – Be humble
82. Zvikomborero – Blessing
83. Chengetai – Take care
84. Chipo – Gift
85. Danai – Love one another
86. Gamu – Game
87. Kuda – Love
88. Mudiwa – Beloved
89. Natsai – Be agreeable
90. Nyaradzo – Consolation
91. Panashe – With God
92. Rufaro – Joy
93. Shingirai – Look at
94. Takudzwa – We have been honored
95. Tawanda – We have been multiplied
96. Tendai – Be thankful
97. Tinaye – With God
98. Tonderai – Look at
99. Vongai – Be humble
100. Zviko – Gift

Zambian baby names and their meanings

1. Abigail – Source of Joy
2. Alick – Defender of Mankind
3. Amara – Grace
4. Bwalya – It's a New Day
5. Chanda – Shield
6. Daka – A Dove
7. Efia – Born on Friday
8. Fungai – Think
9. Gondwe – Last Born
10. Hakainde – To Share
11. Imani – Faith
12. Jengo – Building
13. Kaelo – Destiny
14. Langa – Sun
15. Masiye – Accept
16. Nandi – Sweet
17. Oba – King
18. Penda – Love
19. Quoba – Queen
20. Rudo – Love
21. Sampa – Kindness
22. Tandi – Beloved
23. Ulimba – Strength
24. Vuyisile – Joy
25. Wanga – Desire
26. Xola – Stay in Peace
27. Yande – God is Watching
28. Zikomo – Thank You
29. Akani – To Build
30. Bwezani – How are you?
31. Chibwe – Blessing
32. Dalitso – Blessings
33. Esnart – Grace
34. Fungisai – Remember

35. Gamba – Warrior
36. Halima – Gentle
37. Inonge – Gift
38. Jairos – God's Gift
39. Kuda – Love
40. Lunga – Clever
41. Mumba – Creator
42. Nkole – Counsel
43. Obed – Servant
44. Pumulo – Rest
45. Qhawe – Hero
46. Rumbidzai – Praise
47. Simba – Strength
48. Tawonga – We are thankful
49. Uzoma – Good Journey
50. Vimbai – Trust
51. Wako – Your Child
52. Xhanti – Patience
53. Yollanda – Violet Flower
54. Zalika – Well Born
55. Amani – Peace
56. Bongani – Be Thankful
57. Chipo – Gift
58. Dumi – Inspiration
59. Eshe – Life
60. Farai – Rejoice
61. Gwiza – Knowledge
62. Hadija – Early Born
63. Isheanesu – God is with us
64. Jabulani – Rejoice
65. Kundai – Love Each Other
66. Luyando – Love
67. Mwila – Good Luck
68. Nia – Purpose
69. Onani – Look
70. Palesa – Flower

71. Qhubani – Strong
72. Rutendo – Faith
73. Sipho – Gift
74. Thabo – Joy
75. Udo – Peace
76. Vusumuzi – Rebuild the Home
77. Wanjiru – Daughter of a Shepherd
78. Xolani – Peace
79. Yara – Butterfly
80. Zuri – Beautiful
81. Akili – Wisdom
82. Buhle – Beauty
83. Chikondi – Love
84. Daliso – Blessing
85. Esi – Born on Sunday
86. Fadzai – Make Happy
87. Gugu – Precious
88. Hamba – Travel
89. Ife – Love
90. Jengo – Construction
91. Kuziva – Knowing
92. Lombe – Grace
93. Mudiwa – Beloved
94. Nthanda – Star
95. Olwethu – Our Own
96. Pendo – Love
97. Qinisile – Be Strong
98. Ruvimbo – Hope
99. Sibusiso – Blessing
100. Tapiwa – Given

Malawian baby names and their meanings

1. Abiti - Mother
2. Abusa - Teacher
3. Adimu - Rare
4. Agness - Pure, Holy
5. Akuzike - Praise
6. Alinafe - God is with us
7. Alipo - There is more
8. Amal - Hope
9. Amara - Grace
10. Amina - Trustworthy
11. Anafi - He is with us
12. Andiamo - Let's go
13. Andiseni - Do not hate me
14. Angella - Messenger of God
15. Anjiru - The sun
16. Atupele - Let them choose
17. Baina - The one who loves dance
18. Bakhita - Lucky
19. Banda - Family
20. Bingu - Dance
21. Chabwera - He has come back
22. Chalenga - Challenge
23. Chifundo - Mercy
24. Chikondi - Love
25. Chilombo - Beast
26. Chimwemwe - Joy
27. Chipiliro - Hope
28. Chisomo - Grace
29. Dalitso - Blessings
30. Dalo - Born after a brother
31. Dede - Grasshopper
32. Dziko - World
33. Edina - Delight
34. Effie - Well-spoken

35. Elina - Intelligent
36. Esnat - Grace
37. Fatsani - Be humble
38. Fumbani - Learn
39. Gome - Drum
40. Hara - Be energetic
41. Imani - Faith
42. Ine - Me
43. Jamila - Beautiful
44. Kambiri - Countless
45. Kando - Love
46. Kapeni - Captain
47. Kondwani - Be happy
48. Kukonda - To love
49. Lekeleni - Leave her alone
50. Limbani - Be strong
51. Lina - Tender
52. Lughano - Story
53. Madalitso - Blessings
54. Malia - Of the sea or bitter
55. Mapenzi - Love
56. Masina - Moon
57. Maua - Flower
58. Mbali - Flower
59. Mbekeani - Welcome him
60. Mphatso - Gift
61. Mtima - Heart
62. Mwai - Luck
63. Mwana - Child
64. Namalenga - Creator
65. Nandi - Sweet
66. Nasi - Here
67. Ndale - Issues
68. Nia - Purpose
69. Nthanda - Star
70. Nyalimuzi - Interpreter

71. Nyasa - Lake
72. Pemphero - Prayer
73. Pili - Second
74. Rudo - Love
75. Siti - Lady
76. Tadala - We have been blessed
77. Taonga - We are thankful
78. Tapiwa - Given
79. Tayani - Let's dance
80. Thoko - Praise
81. Tiyamike - Let's praise
82. Ulemu - Respect
83. Wanga - Mine
84. Wokondedwa - Beloved
85. Yankho - Answer
86. Yohane - God is gracious
87. Zalika - Well-born
88. Zikomo - Thank you
89. Zione - It's good
90. Zondiwe - Be saved
91. Zuwa - Sun
92. Zuwena - Good
93. Lusungu - White
94. Mphatso - Gift
95. Mzondi - From the mountain
96. Tionge - Let's tell them
97. Chikumbutso - Memory
98. Chisomo - Favor
99. Dalitso - Blessing
100. Chikondi - Love

Mozambican baby names and their meanings

1. Adelino - Noble
2. Aida - Happy
3. Alcinda - Strong-willed
4. Amadeu - Love of God
5. Amélia - Industrious
6. Aníbal - Grace of Baal
7. Antonia - Priceless
8. Artur - Noble and courageous
9. Berta - Bright and shining
10. Beatriz - Bringer of joy
11. Cândido - Pure
12. Carla - Free woman
13. Catarina - Pure
14. Celestino - Heavenly
15. Cristina - Follower of Christ
16. Damião - To tame
17. Daniela - God is my judge
18. Duarte - Prosperous guardian
19. Elisa - God's promise
20. Ema - Universal
21. Fabio - Bean grower
22. Fernanda - Adventurous
23. Filipe - Lover of horses
24. Gabriela - God's strength
25. Hélder - Respectable
26. Helena - Light
27. Ilda - Battle woman
28. Inês - Pure
29. Joana - God's gracious gift
30. Joaquim - Established by God
31. Jorge - Farmer
32. José - God will add
33. Juliana - Youthful

34. Lúcia - Light
35. Luís - Famous warrior
36. Madalena - Of Magdala
37. Manuel - God is with us
38. Mariana - Grace
39. Marta - Lady
40. Mateus - Gift of God
41. Nuno - Ninth
42. Octávio - Eighth
43. Olga - Holy
44. Patrícia - Noble
45. Paula - Small
46. Quirino - Spear
47. Rafaela - God has healed
48. Ramiro - Wise protector
49. Ricardo - Powerful ruler
50. Rosa - Rose
51. Sílvia - Forest
52. Teresa - Harvester
53. Úrsula - Little bear
54. Valéria - To be strong
55. Vanessa - Butterfly
56. Verónica - True image
57. Xavier - New house
58. Zara - Princess
59. Abel - Breath
60. Adão - Earth
61. Bela - Beautiful
62. César - Long-haired
63. Dinis - God of wine
64. Elói - Chosen
65. Fátima - Captivating
66. Graça - Grace
67. Hugo - Mind, intellect
68. Íris - Rainbow
69. Júlio - Youthful

70. Lara - Cheerful
71. Mafalda - Powerful battler
72. Nádia - Hope
73. Óscar - Divine spear
74. Priscila - Ancient
75. Querubim - Cherub
76. Rúben - Behold, a son
77. Sofia - Wisdom
78. Telma - Will, volition
79. Uriel - God is my light
80. Vitor - Conqueror
81. Xénia - Hospitality
82. Yara - Water lady
83. Zé - God will add
84. Abraão - Father of many
85. Benedito - Blessed
86. Cláudio - Lame
87. Domingos - Belonging to the Lord
88. Estêvão - Crown
89. Felícia - Lucky
90. Guilherme - Resolute protector
91. Ismael - God will hear
92. Jacinta - Hyacinth
93. Leandro - Lion man
94. Micaela - Who is like God?
95. Norberto - Bright north
96. Ofélia - Help
97. Prudêncio - Prudent
98. Quintino - Fifth
99. Raimundo - Wise protector
100. Sebastião - Venerable

Sudanese baby names and their meanings

1. Abayomi - 'Bringer of joy'
2. Adil - 'Just, fair'
3. Aisha - 'Living, prosperous'
4. Akiki - 'Friendly, welcoming'
5. Akol - 'Someone who can be relied on'
6. Alakiir - 'Rainbow'
7. Amal - 'Hope'
8. Amina - 'Trustworthy, faithful'
9. Amira - 'Princess'
10. Anwar - 'Luminous, enlightened'
11. Arif - 'Knowledgeable'
12. Asma - 'Supreme'
13. Ata - 'Gift'
14. Aziza - 'Precious, cherished'
15. Badr - 'Full moon'
16. Bahri - 'Of the sea'
17. Baraka - 'Blessing'
18. Bashir - 'Bearer of good news'
19. Bilal - 'Water, freshness'
20. Bulus - 'Humble, modest'
21. Dalia - 'Gentle'
22. Dina - 'Judged, vindicated'
23. Eiman - 'Faith'
24. Fadil - 'Generous, honorable'
25. Faisal - 'Decisive'
26. Fatima - 'Captivating, a daughter of the Prophet'
27. Gisma - 'Mystery, secret'
28. Habib - 'Beloved'
29. Hadiya - 'Gift'
30. Hafsa - 'Gathering'
31. Hakim - 'Wise'
32. Halima - 'Gentle, patient'
33. Hamza - 'Strong, steadfast'
34. Hassan - 'Handsome, good'

35. Huda - 'Guidance to the right path'
36. Ibrahim - 'Father of multitude'
37. Idris - 'Interpreter'
38. Iman - 'Faith, belief'
39. Isra - 'Nocturnal journey'
40. Jamal - 'Beauty'
41. Jamila - 'Beautiful'
42. Jibril - 'God is my strength'
43. Kamil - 'Perfect'
44. Karim - 'Generous, noble'
45. Khalid - 'Eternal'
46. Khadija - 'Premature child'
47. Layla - 'Night'
48. Lina - 'Tender'
49. Luqman - 'Wise'
50. Maha - 'Wild cow'
51. Mahir - 'Skilled'
52. Majdi - 'Glorious'
53. Malak - 'Angel'
54. Malik - 'King'
55. Mariam - 'Bitter'
56. Marwa - 'Quartz'
57. Mohamed - 'Praiseworthy'
58. Mona - 'Desire, wish'
59. Munir - 'Illuminating, shedding light'
60. Musa - 'Saved from the water'
61. Nabil - 'Noble'
62. Nadia - 'Caller'
63. Nafisa - 'Precious gem'
64. Najwa - 'Secret conversation'
65. Nasir - 'Helper'
66. Nour - 'Light'
67. Omar - 'Long-lived'
68. Rabia - 'Spring'
69. Rashid - 'Rightly guided'
70. Rania - 'Gazing upon'

71. Rasha - 'Young gazelle'
72. Reem - 'Gazelle'
73. Sabir - 'Patient'
74. Saif - 'Sword'
75. Salim - 'Safe, sound'
76. Samira - 'Companion in evening conversation'
77. Sana - 'Radiance, brilliance'
78. Sara - 'Princess'
79. Sharif - 'Noble, honorable'
80. Sumaya - 'High above'
81. Taha - 'Pure'
82. Tariq - 'Morning star'
83. Thabit - 'Firm'
84. Umar - 'Life'
85. Wafiq - 'Successful'
86. Wajdi - 'Passionate'
87. Yasir - 'Wealthy'
88. Yasmin - 'Jasmine flower'
89. Yusra - 'Prosperity'
90. Zafir - 'Victorious'
91. Zahra - 'Flowering, shining'
92. Zain - 'Beauty, grace'
93. Zaki - 'Pure'
94. Zaynab - 'Fragrant flower'
95. Zuhair - 'Bright, shining'
96. Zuhal - 'Saturn'
97. Rasha - 'Young gazelle'
98. Suleiman - 'Man of peace'
99. Tawfiq - 'Success, reconciliation'
100. Yumna - 'Good fortune'

Egyptian baby names and their meanings

1. Aaliyah - High, exalted
2. Abasi - Serious
3. Adio - Righteous
4. Akila - Intelligent
5. Amun - The hidden one
6. Anippe - Daughter of the Nile
7. Asim - Protector
8. Aziza - Precious
9. Badru - Born during the full moon
10. Bahiti - Fortune
11. Bakari - Promise
12. Basim - Smiling
13. Bastet - She of the ointment jar
14. Dalila - Gentle
15. Dua - Worship
16. Eshe - Life
17. Femi - Love me
18. Gamal - Beauty
19. Hasina - Good
20. Heba - Gift from God
21. Isis - Throne
22. Jabari - Brave
23. Jahi - Dignified
24. Kamilah - Perfect
25. Keket - Goddess of darkness
26. Layla - Born at night
27. Maat - Truth, law
28. Maha - Wild cow, beauty
29. Malik - King
30. Naeem - Comfort, ease
31. Nefertiti - Beautiful woman has come
32. Osiris - God of the dead
33. Qabil - Able
34. Ra - Sun

35. Rashida - Righteous
36. Safiya - Pure
37. Shani - Marvelous
38. Tahir - Pure, clean
39. Umm - Mother
40. Zahi - Bright, shining
41. Zuberi - Strong
42. Zula - Brilliant, ahead
43. Afia - Born on Friday
44. Akhenaten - Effective for Aten
45. Anubis - God of death
46. Aten - Sun disk
47. Cairo - Victorious
48. Cleopatra - Glory of the father
49. Djoser - Sacred
50. Edfu - Where Horus is extolled
51. Giza - Hewn stone
52. Hapi - God of the Nile
53. Imhotep - He who comes in peace
54. Kephera - The sun at dawn
55. Luxor - Palaces
56. Menes - The enduring one
57. Nekhbet - She of Nekheb
58. Osorkon - Powerful Osiris
59. Ptah - Creator
60. Ramses - Born of Ra
61. Sekhmet - Powerful woman
62. Thutmose - Born of Thoth
63. Unas - He is strong
64. Zoser - Sacred
65. Amenhotep - Amun is satisfied
66. Astarte - Goddess of war and sexual love
67. Buto - Goddess of the north
68. Hathor - House of Horus
69. Meretseger - She who loves silence
70. Neith - Divine mother

71.	Pakhet -	She who scratches
72.	Qadesh -	Sacred
73.	Serket -	She who causes the throat to breathe
74.	Taweret -	The great female
75.	Wadjet -	Green one
76.	Xois -	Little town
77.	Yamm -	Sea
78.	Zalika -	Well-born
79.	Horus -	God of the sky
80.	Seth -	God of chaos
81.	Nefer -	Beauty, goodness
82.	Djed -	Stability
83.	Maahes -	Lion
84.	Khonsu -	Traveller
85.	Montu -	God of war
86.	Shu -	Emptiness
87.	Geb -	Earth
88.	Nut -	Sky
89.	Heka -	Magic
90.	Wepwawet -	Opener of the ways
91.	Khnum -	Creator
92.	Anhur -	Sky bearer
93.	Sobek -	Crocodile
94.	Min -	God of fertility
95.	Iah -	Moon
96.	Nekhbet -	Vulture goddess
97.	Seshat -	Goddess of writing
98.	Tefnut -	Moisture
99.	Hetepheres -	Her peace is upon her
100.	Ankhesenamun -	Her life is of Amun

Libyan baby names and their meanings

1. Aisha – Living, prosperous
2. Amal – Hope, aspiration
3. Ahmed – Praiseworthy
4. Ali – Exalted, noble
5. Ayoub – Patient
6. Amira – Princess
7. Badr – Full moon
8. Bilal – Water
9. Bahija – Joyful, happy
10. Basim – Smiling
11. Dalia – Grape vine
12. Dina – Judged, vindicated
13. Eman – Faith
14. Fadil – Generous, honorable
15. Farah – Joy, happiness
16. Farid – Unique, precious
17. Fathi – Conqueror
18. Ghada – Graceful, young girl
19. Hadi – Guide to righteousness
20. Hafsa – Young lioness
21. Hakim – Wise, judicious
22. Idris – Studious person
23. Iman – Faith, belief
24. Jamal – Beauty
25. Jannah – Paradise, garden
26. Kamil – Perfect
27. Karima – Generous, noble
28. Khalid – Eternal, immortal
29. Layla – Night
30. Lina – Palm tree
31. Malik – King
32. Mariam – Sea of bitterness, rebelliousness
33. Nabil – Noble, generous
34. Nadia – Caller, announcer

35. Omar – Long-lived
36. Qasim – Divider, distributor
37. Rabia – Spring, fourth female
38. Radwan – Pleasure, satisfaction
39. Saad – Good luck
40. Sabah – Morning
41. Samira – Companion in evening conversation
42. Tariq – Morning star
43. Umar – Life, long living
44. Wafa – Loyalty, faithfulness
45. Yasmine – Jasmine flower
46. Zahra – Flower, blossom
47. Zainab – Fragrant flower
48. Ziad – Abundance, growth
49. Adel – Just, fair
50. Amina – Trustworthy, faithful
51. Aziz – Powerful, beloved
52. Bashar – Bringer of glad tidings
53. Daud – Beloved
54. Esam – Safeguard
55. Faisal – Decisive
56. Fatima – Daughter of the Prophet
57. Galal – Greatness, pride
58. Hana – Happiness
59. Isra – Night journey
60. Jafar – Stream
61. Kamal – Perfection
62. Leila – Night
63. Majed – Noble, glorious
64. Naim – Comfort, tranquility
65. Nour – Light
66. Osama – Lion
67. Rania – Gazing upon
68. Salim – Safe, sound
69. Taha – Pure
70. Uthman – Baby bustard

71. Yasir – Wealthy
72. Zafir – Victorious
73. Zuhair – Bright, shining
74. Asma – High, exalted
75. Baha – Splendor, glory
76. Dalal – Treated or touched in a kind and loving way
77. Elham – Inspiration
78. Fadi – Redeemer
79. Ghassan – Youth, prime of life
80. Hisham – Generous
81. Jamal – Beauty
82. Khaled – Immortal
83. Lulu – Pearl
84. Maged – Praiseworthy
85. Nada – Generosity, dew
86. Nizar – Little
87. Othman – Companion of the Prophet
88. Rasha – Young gazelle
89. Sabri – Patient
90. Tawfik – Success, reconciliation
91. Wahid – Unique
92. Yara – Small butterfly
93. Zain – Grace, beauty
94. Asaad – Happiest
95. Basma – Smile
96. Dounia – The world
97. Fawzi – Successful
98. Ghalia – Precious
99. Hashem – Crusher, breaker
100. Jamila – Beautiful

Algerian baby names and their meanings

1. Aasiyah - 'consoling' or 'comforting'
2. Abdul - Servant of God
3. Amina - Trustworthy and faithful
4. Amira - Princess
5. Ali - Exalted, noble
6. Aicha - Alive
7. Bilal - Water, freshness
8. Bouchra - The one who is good
9. Chafik - Sympathetic
10. Dalila - Guide, model
11. Djamila - Beautiful
12. Fadila - Virtuous
13. Farid - Unique, precious
14. Fatima - Captivating
15. Ghani - Rich, wealthy
16. Hakim - Wise, judicious
17. Hassan - Handsome, good
18. Hafsa - Young lioness
19. Idris - Studious, knowledgeable
20. Imene - Faith, belief
21. Jamila - Beautiful
22. Kader - Powerful, capable
23. Karim - Generous
24. Khadija - First wife of Prophet Muhammad
25. Lamine - Trustworthy
26. Leila - Night
27. Malika - Queen
28. Mohamed - Praised, commendable
29. Nabila - Noble, honorable
30. Nadia - Caller, announcer
31. Omar - Long-lived
32. Rabia - Spring
33. Sabrina - From the river Severn
34. Samira - Companion in evening conversation

35. Tariq - Morning star
36. Yasmina - Jasmine flower
37. Zahra - Bright, shining
38. Zainab - Fragrant flower
39. Zohra - Venus, beauty
40. Zoulikha - Beautiful
41. Faisal - Strong, handsome
42. Yasmine - Jasmine flower
43. Nadir - Rare, precious
44. Rania - Queen
45. Salim - Safe, healthy
46. Souad - Happiness, luck
47. Taha - Pure
48. Wafa - Loyalty
49. Yacine - Rich, prosperous
50. Zineb - Good, beautiful
51. Aamir - Civilized, abundant
52. Bahija - Joyful, happy
53. Chahine - Falcon
54. Dounia - World, life
55. Elias - The Lord is my God
56. Fathi - Conqueror
57. Ghizlane - Gazelle
58. Houda - Guidance to the right path
59. Imane - Faith
60. Jalila - Great, revered
61. Kamel - Perfect
62. Latifa - Gentle, kind
63. Mounir - Shining, luminous
64. Naima - Comfort, tranquility
65. Oussama - Lion
66. Rafik - Friend, companion
67. Saida - Happy, fortunate
68. Tahar - Pure, chaste
69. Wahiba - Giver
70. Youssef - God will add

71. Zakaria - God has remembered
72. Aicha - Living, prosperous
73. Badr - Full moon
74. Chaima - With a beauty spot
75. Djamel - Beauty
76. Fares - Knight, horseman
77. Halima - Gentle, patient
78. Ismail - God will hear
79. Jamel - Handsome
80. Karima - Generous, noble
81. Leila - Night
82. Malika - Queen
83. Nour - Light
84. Othman - Baby bustard
85. Rachid - Rightly guided
86. Samia - Elevated, sublime
87. Tarek - Morning star
88. Wahid - Unique, singular
89. Yara - Small butterfly
90. Zahir - Bright, shining
91. Amine - Trustworthy, faithful
92. Basma - Smile
93. Cherif - Noble, distinguished
94. Dalia - Branch, vine
95. Elina - Intelligent
96. Fathiya - Conqueror
97. Habiba - Beloved, sweetheart
98. Iman - Faith, belief
99. Jalal - Majesty, greatness
100. Kamila - Perfect

Tunisian baby names and their meanings

1. Aaliyah - Exalted, highest social standing
2. Abir - Fragrance, perfume
3. Adam - The first human
4. Adel - Just, fair
5. Afif - Chaste, modest
6. Ahlam - Dreams
7. Aicha - Alive, well
8. Akram - Most generous
9. Alia - Exalted, noble
10. Amal - Hope
11. Amine - Faithful, trustworthy
12. Anis - Friendly, companion
13. Asma - Supreme, excellent
14. Aya - Miracle, sign
15. Ayman - Blessed, lucky
16. Badr - Full moon
17. Bahija - Joyful, happy
18. Basim - Smiling
19. Bilal - Water, moisture
20. Chaima - With a beauty spot
21. Dalila - Guide, model
22. Dalia - Vine, branch
23. Dhafer - Victorious
24. Elham - Inspiration
25. Emna - Faithful, to believe
26. Eya - Beautiful eyes
27. Fadhel - Virtuous, superior
28. Fadia - Saviour
29. Fadwa - Self-sacrifice
30. Fares - Knight
31. Farid - Unique, singular
32. Fatma - One who abstains
33. Firas - Perspicacity
34. Ghada - Graceful, young girl

35. Ghofran - Forgiveness, pardon
36. Habib - Beloved
37. Hafsa - Young lioness
38. Hakim - Wise, judicious
39. Halima - Gentle, patient
40. Hamza - Strong, steadfast
41. Hanan - Mercy, compassion
42. Hedi - Leader, guide
43. Houda - Right guidance
44. Ibtissem - Smile
45. Idris - Studious, learned
46. Imen - Faith, belief
47. Ines - Pure, holy
48. Issam - Safeguard
49. Jamila - Beautiful
50. Jihen - Universe
51. Kais - Firm, hard
52. Karim - Generous, noble
53. Khaled - Eternal
54. Lamia - Radiant, brilliant
55. Leila - Night
56. Lina - Tender, delicate
57. Lotfi - Kind, gentle
58. Maha - Wild cow, deer
59. Majed - Glorious
60. Malak - Angel
61. Marwa - A fragrant plant
62. Medhi - Guided one
63. Meriem - Beloved, wished-for child
64. Moez - Honorable
65. Monia - Wish, desire
66. Nabil - Noble, generous
67. Nadia - Caller, announcer
68. Naim - Comfort, tranquility
69. Nawel - Gift
70. Nizar - Little, rare

71. Noor - Light
72. Oussama - Lion
73. Rachid - Rightly guided
74. Rafik - Friend, companion
75. Rania - Gazing upon
76. Rayan - Watered, luxuriant
77. Riadh - Gardens
78. Rym - Gazelle
79. Saber - Patient
80. Salim - Safe, sound
81. Sami - High, exalted
82. Samir - Entertaining companion
83. Selim - Safe, sound
84. Sihem - Arrow
85. Skander - Defender of mankind
86. Sofiene - Devoted
87. Sonia - Gold
88. Tarek - Morning star
89. Thouraya - Pleiades star cluster
90. Wafa - Faithfulness
91. Walid - Newborn
92. Wassim - Handsome
93. Yasmine - Jasmine flower
94. Yosra - Ease, comfort
95. Youssef - God will add
96. Zainab - Father's joy
97. Zied - Growth, increase
98. Ziyad - Abundance, growth
99. Zohra - Blooming, shining
100. Zouhair - Small flower

Christian Names

Adam - "Man of the earth" or "to be red"
Eve - "Living" or "life"
Noah - "Rest" or "comfort"
Sarah - "Princess" or "lady"
Abraham - "Father of many" or "father of a multitude"
Rebekah - "To tie" or "to bind"
Isaac - "He laughs" or "laughter"
Rachel - "Ewe" or "female sheep"
Jacob - "Supplanter" or "one who grabs the heel"
Leah - "Weary" or "tired"
Joseph - "May God add" or "God will increase"
Mary - "Bitter" or "beloved"
Jesus - "God saves" or "Yahweh saves"
John - "God is gracious"
Peter - "Rock" or "stone"
Paul - "Small" or "humble"
Luke - "Light-giving" or "from Lucania"
Mark - "Warlike" or "consecrated to Mars"
Matthew - "Gift of God"
Timothy - "Honoring God" or "to honor God"
Andrew - "Manly" or "brave"
David - "Beloved" or "friend"
Hannah - "Grace" or "favor"
Samuel - "Name of God" or "God has heard"
Esther - "Star" or "myrtle leaf"
Solomon - "Peace" or "peaceful"
Deborah - "Bee" or "bee-like"
Ruth - "Companion" or "friend"
Daniel - "God is my judge"
Gabriel - "God is my strength" or "man of God"
Michael - "Who is like God?"
Raphael - "God heals"
Elijah - "My God is Yahweh" or "Yahweh is God"
Joshua - "Yahweh is salvation"

Ruth - "Friendship" or "companion"
Naomi - "Pleasantness" or "sweetness"
Daniel - "God is my judge"
Rebecca - "To tie" or "to bind"
Hannah - "Favor" or "grace"
Gideon - "Feller" or "hewer"
Deborah - "Bee" or "honeybee"
Abigail - "Father's joy" or "source of joy"
Timothy - "Honoring God" or "to honor God"
Tabitha - "Gazelle" or "deer"
Jonathan - "God has given" or "gift of God"
Martha - "Lady" or "mistress"
Mary - "Sea of bitterness" or "rebelliousness"
Lazarus - "God has helped" or "God is my help"
Jacob - "Supplanter" or "holder of the heel"
Rebecca - "To tie" or "to bind"
Deborah - "Bee" or "honeybee"
Esther - "Star" or "myrtle leaf"
Joshua - "Yahweh is salvation"
Naomi - "Pleasantness" or "sweetness"
Samuel - "Name of God" or "God has heard"
Solomon - "Peace" or "peaceful"
Anna - "Grace" or "favor"
Abigail - "Father's joy" or "source of joy"
Elijah - "My God is Yahweh" or "Yahweh is God"
Rachel - "Ewe" or "female sheep"
Sarah - "Princess" or "lady"
Caleb - "Dog" or "faithful"
Elizabeth - "God is my oath" or "God's promise"
Daniel - "God is my judge"
Aaron - "Exalted" or "high mountain"
Jacob - "Supplanter" or "holder of the heel"
Hannah - "Favor" or "grace"
Matthew - "Gift of God"
James - "Supplanter" or "one who follows"
Levi - "Joined" or "attached"

Ruth - "Friendship" or "companion"
Lydia - "From Lydia" or "woman from Lydia"
Phoebe - "Bright" or "radiant"
Caleb - "Dog" or "faithful"
Miriam - "Sea of bitterness" or "rebelliousness"
Benjamin - "Son of the right hand" or "son of the south"
Joel - "Yahweh is God"
Silas - "Of the forest" or "wood-dweller"
Aaron - "Exalted" or "high mountain"
Tabitha - "Gazelle" or "deer"
Levi - "Joined" or "attached"
Matthias - "Gift of Yahweh"
Stephen - "Crown" or "garland"
Philip - "Lover of horses" or "friend of horses"
Barnabas - "Son of encouragement"
Nathaniel - "Gift of God"
Seth - "Appointed" or "placed"
Luke - "Light-giving" or "from Lucania"
Nathan - "He gave" or "gift from God"
Tobias - "God is good" or "Yahweh is good"
Jonathan - "God has given" or "gift of God"
Amos - "Burden" or "burden-bearer"
Timothy - "Honoring God" or "to honor God"
Silas - "Of the forest" or "wood-dweller"
Barnabas - "Son of encouragement"
Nathaniel - "Gift of God"
Seth - "Appointed" or "placed"
Ezra - "Help" or "helper"
Asa - "Healer" or "physician"
Micah - "Who is like Yahweh?" or "Who is like God?"

Islamic Names

Bilal - "Moisture" or "freshness"
Khalid - "Eternal" or "immortal"
Musa - "Drawn out" or "saved from water"
Malik - "King" or "sovereign"
Jamal - "Beauty" or "grace"
Yasmine - "Jasmine flower" or "fragrant flower"
Ilyas - "Prophet Elijah" or "the Lord is my God"
Omar - "Flourishing" or "long-lived"
Sulaiman - "Man of peace" or "peaceful"
Amina - "Trustworthy" or "faithful"
Rahim - "Merciful" or "kind"
Zakariya - "Remembered by God" or "God remembers"
Adil - "Just" or "fair"
Hassan - "Good" or "handsome"
Tariq - "Morning star" or "he who knocks at the door"
Rania - "Content" or "satisfied"
Kareem - "Generous" or "noble"
Latifah - "Kind" or "gentle"
Farid - "Unique" or "precious"
Samira - "Companion in evening talk" or "pleasant community"

Hindu Names

Aarav - "Peaceful" or "wise"
Aadya - "First" or "original"
Aarushi - "First rays of the sun" or "first light"
Aditi - "Boundless" or "limitless"
Advik - "Unique" or "one of a kind"
Aisha - "Alive" or "prosperous"
Anaya - "Unique" or "different"
Anika - "Goddess Durga" or "grace"
Arjun - "Bright" or "shining"
Ayush - "Long life" or "ageless"
Bhavya - "Grand" or "splendid"
Dhruv - "Constant" or "steadfast"
Divya - "Divine" or "heavenly"
Esha - "Desire" or "wish"
Ishaan - "Lord Shiva" or "sun"
Kavya - "Poetry" or "poem"
Kiara - "Dark-haired" or "little dark one"
Krish - "Short form of Krishna" or "attractive"
Maya - "Illusion" or "magic"
Neel - "Blue" or "sapphire"
Riya - "Singer" or "melody"
Rishi - "Sage" or "saint"
Riyaan - "Door of heaven" or "paradise"
Saanvi - "Goddess Lakshmi" or "knowledge"
Siddharth - "One who has achieved his goal" or "enlightened"
Tanisha - "Ambition" or "desire"
Yash - "Fame" or "glory"
Advait - "Unique" or "one of a kind"
Akshara - "Imperishable" or "indestructible"
Arya - "Noble" or "honorable"
Dhruv - "Pole star" or "steadfast"
Isha - "Desire" or "wish"
Jiya - "Heart" or "soul"

Kaira - "Peaceful" or "unique"
Kian - "Grace of God" or "king"
Krish - "Short form of Krishna" or "attractive"
Meera - "Ocean" or "boundary"
Neil - "Champion" or "cloud"
Nirav - "Quiet" or "silent"
Oviya - "Artist" or "beautiful drawing"
Parth - "Prince" or "son of Pritha"
Reyansh - "Ray of light" or "part of God"
Rohan - "Ascending" or "growing"
Saanvi - "Goddess Lakshmi" or "knowledge"
Shreya - "Fortunate" or "auspicious"
Tanvi - "Goddess of beauty" or "slender"
Ved - "Knowledge" or "sacred knowledge"
Vihaan - "Dawn" or "morning"
Aarav - "Peaceful" or "wise"
Aadya - "First" or "original"
Anika - "Goddess Durga" or "grace"
Arjun - "Bright" or "shining"
Ayush - "Long life" or "ageless"
Dhruv - "Constant" or "steadfast"
Divya - "Divine" or "heavenly"
Esha - "Desire" or "wish"
Ishaan - "Lord Shiva" or "sun"
Kavya - "Poetry" or "poem"
Kiara - "Dark-haired" or "little dark one"
Maya - "Illusion" or "magic"
Neel - "Blue" or "sapphire"
Riya - "Singer" or "melody"
Rishi - "Sage" or "saint"
Riyaan - "Door of heaven" or "paradise"
Siddharth - "One who has achieved his goal" or "enlightened"
Tanisha - "Ambition" or "desire"
Yash - "Fame" or "glory"
Akshara - "Imperishable" or "indestructible"

Arya - "Noble" or "honorable"
Isha - "Desire" or "wish"

Buddhist Names

Bodhi - "Awakening" or "enlightenment"
Dharma - "The path" or "the teachings of the Buddha"
Ashoka - "Without sorrow" or "without worry"
Kaya - "Body" or "physical form"
Tara - "Star" or "goddess of compassion"
Zen - "Meditation" or "absorption"
Ananda - "Bliss" or "happiness"
Surya - "Sun" or "solar deity"
Sangha - "Community" or "assembly of followers"
Deva - "God" or "divine being"
Jaya - "Victory" or "triumph"
Karuna - "Compassion" or "mercy"
Metta - "Loving-kindness" or "benevolence"
Virya - "Energy" or "vigor"
Nirvana - "Liberation" or "enlightenment"
Maya - "Illusion" or "magic"
Sati - "Mindfulness" or "awareness"
Samsara - "Cycle of existence" or "worldly life"
Bodhisattva - "Enlightened being" or "awakened being"
Anicca - "Impermanence" or "transience"
Jhana - "Meditative absorption" or "deep concentration"
Panna - "Wisdom" or "insight"
Kshanti - "Patience" or "endurance"
Satya - "Truth" or "truthfulness"
Bhavana - "Mental development" or "cultivation"
Upasaka - "Lay follower" or "devotee"
Samadhi - "Concentration" or "meditative absorption"
Sutra - "Scripture" or "sacred text"
Nanda - "Joy" or "delight"
Sila - "Ethical conduct" or "morality"

Bodhisara - "Aspiring Bodhisattva" or "seeker of enlightenment"
Arhat - "Worthy one" or "enlightened being"
Abhaya - "Fearless" or "without fear"
Karunika - "Compassionate" or "merciful"

Jewish Names

Aaron - "High mountain" or "exalted"
Leah - "Weary" or "tired"
Isaac - "He will laugh" or "laughter"
Hannah - "Grace" or "favor"
Jacob - "Supplanter" or "holder of the heel"
Sarah - "Princess" or "noblewoman"
Joshua - "The Lord is salvation" or "God rescues"
Rachel - "Ewe" or "female sheep"
David - "Beloved" or "friend"
Miriam - "Sea of bitterness" or "rebelliousness"
Benjamin - "Son of the right hand" or "son of the south"
Rebecca - "To bind" or "to tie"
Samuel - "Name of God" or "God has heard"
Esther - "Star" or "myrtle leaf"
Solomon - "Peace" or "peaceful"
Ruth - "Companion" or "friend"
Ezekiel - "God will strengthen" or "God will harden"
Judith - "Jewish woman" or "woman from Judea"
Daniel - "God is my judge" or "God is my strength"
Abigail - "My father's joy" or "source of joy"
Isaiah - "Salvation of the Lord" or "God is salvation"
Deborah - "Bee" or "honey bee"
Nathan - "He gave" or "gift of God"

Sikh Names

Ajeet - "Invincible"
Gurpreet - "Love of the Guru"
Harman - "Beloved"
Jasleen - "Absorbed in singing praises of the Lord"
Manpreet - "One who loves the mind of the Almighty"
Navtej - "New light"
Simran - "Remembrance"
Harmanpreet - "Beloved of the Almighty"
Gurleen - "One who is absorbed in the Guru's support"
Ravinder - "Sun"
Manjit - "Victorious"
Harpreet - "Love of the Almighty"
Tejinder - "Radiant God"
Amardeep - "Eternal light"
Kirpal - "Compassionate"
Jaskiran - "Rays of the Lord's light"
Jasbir - "Brave"
Jagdeep - "Light of the universe"
Navjot - "New light"
Simarjeet - "Victory by remembering God"
Harvinder - "Lord's presence"
Gurcharan - "Feet of the Guru"
Satnam - "True name"
Harjinder - "Victory of the Almighty"
Kiranpreet - "One who loves the rays of the sun"

Millennial Baby Names

Girls:
Emma, Olivia, Sophia, Ava, Isabella, Mia, Abigail, Emily, Madison, Charlotte, Harper, Amelia, Evelyn, Elizabeth, Sofia, Avery, Ella, Scarlett, Grace, Lily, Aria, Chloe, Zoey, Penelope, Layla, Riley, Nora, Harper, Zoe, Lillian, Natalie, Hannah, Aubrey, Adalyn, Stella, Taylor, Victoria, Evelyn, Samantha, Skylar, Alexa, Alexis, Claire, Peyton, Leah, Lucy, Bella, Audrey, Savannah, Allison, Elena, Madelyn, Gabriella, Ruby, Kaylee, Eva, Madeline, Kinsley, Autumn, Faith, Emilia, Annabelle, Aaliyah, Caroline, Kennedy, Ellie, Hazel, Violet, Cora, Jasmine, Nina, Isabelle, Maya, Ariana, Maria, Sophie, Brielle, Mackenzie, Kennedy, Luna, Peyton, Rose, Nova, Trinity, Lila, Bella, Sienna, Mary, Georgia, Elise, Holly, Melody, Valerie, Brianna, Everly, Laila, Angelina, Fiona, Angela, Giselle, Daniela, Amaya, Leilani, Jade, Rebecca, Juliana, Alaina, Esther, Margaret, Laura, Alexis, Eloise, Paige, Harmony, Jane, Alma, Bianca, Lydia, Ruth, Annie, Mabel, Olive, Danielle, Clara, Sarah, Hope, Phoebe, Reese, Mya, Jennifer, Adriana, Everleigh, Joy, Arabella, Heidi, Tessa, Lyla, Mackenzie, Willow, Annalise, Amara, Ariel, Lana, Veronic

Boys:
Liam, Noah, Ethan, Mason, Logan, Lucas, Jackson, Aiden, Oliver, Elijah, Alexander, James, Benjamin, Jacob, William, Michael, Daniel, Henry, Owen, Samuel, Sebastian, David, Carter, Matthew, Joseph, Julian, Isaac, Gabriel, Wyatt, Anthony, Andrew, John, Christopher, Joshua, Nathan, Isaac, Jonathan, Evan, Aaron, Cameron, Christian, Colton, Landon, Nicholas, Connor, Jeremiah, Josiah, Adrian, Leo, Hudson, Robert, Angel, Brayden, Gavin, Dominic, Austin, Jordan, Lincoln, Adam, Ian, Elias, Thomas, Christopher,

Xavier, Zachary, Nolan, Max, Samuel, Chase, Cole, Brody, Grayson, Oscar, Tyler, Parker, Ryder, Diego, Luis, Wesley, Kai, Jace, Finn, Emmett, Harrison, Roman, Bennett, George, Miles, Jasper, Leonardo, Julian, Asher, Levi, Theodore, Nathaniel

1950s Baby Names

Girls:
Mary, Linda, Patricia, Susan, Deborah, Barbara, Sandra, Nancy, Karen, Donna, Carol, Sharon, Brenda, Diane, Pamela, Kathleen, Cheryl, Elizabeth, Janet, Cynthia, Judith, Judy, Kathy, Joan, Betty, Joyce, Carolyn, Margaret, Beverly, Shirley, Marilyn, Janet, Janet, Bonnie, Diane, Christine, Ann, Jean, Janice, Victoria, Marilyn, Christine, Lois, Phyllis, Kathryn, Martha, Maria, Gail, Marsha, Paula, Marlene, Judith, Joyce, Virginia, Ruth, Norma, Denise, Ellen, Alice, Sylvia, Constance, Frances, Jacqueline, Gloria, Annette, Marjorie, Beatrice, Sue, Elaine, Andrea, Jacqueline, Rita, Rachel, Rose, Marjorie, Louise, Rosemary, Caroline, Rebecca, Lucy, Eileen, Alma, Annette, Paula, Bernice, Lorraine, Maxine, Yvonne, Ella, Bessie, Alberta, Lydia, Loretta, Lillian, Leah, Sarah, Melinda, Irene, Geneva, Doris

Boys:
James, Michael, Robert, John, David, William, Richard, Thomas, Charles, Gary, Larry, Ronald, Donald, Kenneth, Steven, Joseph, Dennis, Daniel, Stephen, George, Edward, Paul, Jerry, Gregory, Bruce, Terry, Timothy, Roger, Ralph, Roy, Carl, Lawrence, Raymond, Arthur, Frank, Harold, Douglas, Wayne, Bobby, Joe, Philip, Eugene, Peter, Russell, Howard, Jeffrey, Clarence, Alan, Gerald, Eugene, Stanley, Jesse, Norman, Samuel, Phillip, Johnny, Billy, Allen, Glenn, Willie, Jack, Louis, Leonard, Gerald, Bruce, Dale, Jay, Rodney, Martin, Ernest, Clarence, Henry, Bobby, Victor, Fred, Steve, Marvin, Bill, Roy, Jesse, Francis, Herbert, Dean, Lloyd, Lee, Leslie, Marvin, Gordon, Arthur, Elmer, Vernon, Melvin, Curtis, Eugene, Karl

1960s Baby Names

Girls:
Mary, Lisa, Susan, Karen, Kimberly, Patricia, Linda, Donna, Michelle, Cynthia, Sandra, Deborah, Tammy, Pamela, Sharon, Angela, Jennifer, Brenda, Laura, Julie, Christine, Elizabeth, Diane, Carolyn, Tracy, Janet, Melissa, Wendy, Kelly, Andrea, Cheryl, Teresa, Robin, Rebecca, Denise, Amy, Dawn, Kathy, Laurie, Stephanie, Tina, Rhonda, Shannon, Carol, Victoria, Cindy, Stacey, Michelle, April, Gina, Ellen, Tonya, Kristine, Leslie, Monica, Jodi, Belinda, Christina, Renee, Jill, Catherine, Sheila, Lori, Carrie, Jamie, Sherry, Beth, Melanie, Shelly, Valerie, Becky, Mindy, Annie, Paula, Regina, Tanya, Carla, Kristin, Vanessa, Tasha, Anne, Janice, Brandy, Rachel, Casey, Tami, Samantha, Joanna, Stacy, Dana, Bobbi, Penny, Kelli, Traci, Cindy, Staci, Summer, Cassandra, Terra, Cari, Angie, Sandy, Debbie

Boys:
Michael, James, David, John, Robert, Mark, William, Richard, Christopher, Brian, Steven, Jeffrey, Timothy, Kevin, Scott, Joseph, Charles, Thomas, Daniel, Anthony, Paul, Kenneth, Gregory, Eric, Stephen, Andrew, Ronald, Patrick, Gary, Douglas, Edward, Todd, Keith, Larry, Shawn, Terry, Dennis, Randy, Jerry, Sean, Peter, Craig, Bradley, Curtis, Russell, Rodney, Allen, Derrick, Phillip, Chad, Rodney, Steve, Tony, Steve, Nathaniel, Curtis, Danny, Billy, Keith, Ryan, Bruce, Rodney, Sean, Tony, Barry, Roger, Philip, Corey, Scott, Roy, Nicholas, Albert, Brandon, Marcus, Ernest, Karl, Chad, Calvin, Vince, Jamie, Brent, Vincent, Roger, Edgar, Dwight, Erik, Theodor

1970s Baby Names

Girls:
Jennifer, Amy, Melissa, Angela, Michelle, Heather, Kimberly, Amanda, Jessica, Nicole, Elizabeth, Sarah, Stephanie, Lisa, Rebecca, Kelly, Christina, Mary, Laura, Jamie, Erin, Rachel, Crystal, Shannon, Megan, Emily, Julie, Tiffany, Christine, Sara, Andrea, Amber, Danielle, Tara, Katie, Monica, Kristin, Allison, Courtney, Veronica, Carly, Candace, Miranda, Natasha, Alicia, Kristy, Jill, Kathryn, Stacey, Renee, Valerie, Karen, Sonia, Trisha, Joanna, Meghan, Carolyn, Tricia, Anna, Tracie, Meredith, Alisa, Jessie, Angelica, Kelli, Bethany, Brittney, Leslie, Janelle, Beth, Marissa, Joanne, Alexis, Sylvia, Brandi, Jacquelyn, Bobbi, Gina, Christy, Misty, Latoya, Chandra, Bobbie, Latasha, Alyssa, Hollie, Adrienne, Sherri, Bianca, Jenna, Leticia, Felicia, Jasmine, Angelina, Alisha, Janice, Shana, Rosanna, Maureen, Jodie, Patrice, Lydia, Ebony, Jaime, Yolanda, Shameka, Susie, Alejandra, Daisy, Tomika, Marisela, Sharonda, Antoinette, Lakisha, Kisha, Lacey, Tiffani, Kenya, Reyna, Araceli

Boys:
Michael, Christopher, Jason, David, James, Matthew, Joshua, John, Robert, Brian, Daniel, Joseph, Ryan, Jeffrey, William, Anthony, Eric, Steven, Kevin, Timothy, Thomas, Richard, Jeremy, Andrew, Brandon, Justin, Nicholas, Gregory, Aaron, Shawn, Benjamin, Scott, Nathan, Charles, Stephen, Travis, Patrick, Kenneth, Paul, Sean, Bryan, Alex, Edward, Keith, Zachary, Mark, Philip, Jared, Dustin, Antonio, Juan, Caleb, Roger, Ian, George, Terry, Jesse, Lawrence, Manuel, Danny, Gerald, Mario, Sergio, Kurt, Randall, Javier, Allan, Brett, Billy, Cody, Harold, Jimmy, Maurice, Frank, Eddie, Rick, Harry, Arnold, Warren, Tommy, Julio, Darren, Rene, Ron, Terrence, Sidney, Glen, Brent, Leo, Alberto, Andy, Terrell, Gilbert, Don, Alvin, Carlton, Stuart,

Ramon, Duane, Elmer, Elvis, Horace, Julius, Vaughn, Leland, Glen, Dana, Ollie, Fredrick, Jayson, Grant, Doug, Blake, Neil, Nolan, Dion, Rickie, Emil, Jesus

1980s Baby Names

Girls:
Jessica, Jennifer, Amanda, Ashley, Sarah, Melissa, Nicole, Stephanie, Heather, Elizabeth, Michelle, Tiffany, Kimberly, Christina, Lauren, Amy, Emily, Samantha, Rachel, Megan, Brittany, Laura, Rebecca, Danielle, Amber, Erin, Erica, Katie, Allison, Anna, Victoria, Crystal, Courtney, Shannon, Lisa, Jamie, Angela, Tara, Kristen, April, Kelly, Lindsey, Andrea, Sara, Katherine, Maria, Brandi, Julie, Alicia, Shannon, Whitney, Cassandra, Valerie, Alicia, Natalie, Valerie, Veronica, Leslie, Adrienne, Caitlin, Monica, Natasha, Marissa, Casey, Sabrina, Kelsey, Denise, Katie, Miranda, Kristin, Desiree, Deanna, Kristina, Felicia, Chelsea, Krista, Holly, Joanna, Carrie, Sylvia, Regina, Trisha, Bethany, Sheri, Jacqueline, Latasha, Misty, Kendra, Kari, Yesenia, Kelli, Kenya, Meghan, Shanna, Ariel, Kristy, Kari, Traci, Latoya, Stacey, Christy, Shana, Brandy, Meagan, Christa, Kristi, Kasey, Keri, Marla, Whitney, Janelle, Tabitha, Lindsey, Angelica, Janine, Angel, Ashleigh, Jami, Leanne, Sonia, Tia, Shelly, Kristie, Danica, Maribel, Clarissa, Misty, Jasmin, Tasha, Jayme, Tanya, Kia, Carrie, Desiree, Mercedes, Marquita, Gwendolyn, Kisha, Shari, Tara, Jasmin, Tameka, Krystal, Brandy, Katelyn, Yvette, Mara, Kyra, Leticia, Janie, Lacie, Christi, Christa, Priscilla, Tricia

Boys:
Michael, Christopher, Matthew, Joshua, David, James, Daniel, Robert, John, Joseph, Ryan, William, Brandon, Jeffrey, Jason, Justin, Brian, Nicholas, Eric, Anthony, Steven, Timothy, Andrew, Kevin, Thomas, Aaron, Richard, Mark, Jonathan, Jeremy, Benjamin, Adam, Charles, Stephen, Scott, Nathan, Patrick, Travis, Kenneth, Kyle, Gregory, Jesse, Sean, Bryan, Edward, Alexander, Paul, Derrick, Cody, Jared, Phillip, Marcus, Zachary, Juan, Bradley, Donald, Gary,

Raymond, Keith, Corey, Shane, Terry, Brett, Roger, Ronald, Todd, Douglas, Curtis, Vincent, Dennis, Derrick, Carlos, Gary, Antonio, Peter, Jerry, Russell, Lawrence, Wesley, Erik, Rodney, Allan, Henry

1990s Baby Names

Girls:

Jessica, Ashley, Emily, Samantha, Sarah, Amanda, Brittany, Taylor, Megan, Nicole, Rachel, Elizabeth, Lauren, Hannah, Victoria, Jennifer, Alyssa, Kayla, Stephanie, Alexandra, Kelsey, Amber, Courtney, Brianna, Danielle, Rebecca, Madison, Michelle, Jasmine, Sydney, Julia, Natalie, Abby, Morgan, Emma, Erin, Allison, Lindsey, Angela, Jenna, Chelsea, Maria, Alexis, Laura, Caitlin, Tiffany, Kelly, Sara, Destiny, Brooke, Cassandra, Katie, Andrea, Mary, Heather, Shelby, Paige, Tara, Caroline, Angelica, Marissa, Christina, Monica, Sierra, Whitney, Veronica, Shannon, Leah, Cassidy, Kristen, Miranda, Valerie, Carly, Claire, Leslie, Mallory, Angel, Alicia, Caitlyn, Audrey, Jamie, Joanne, Dawn, Holly, Jacqueline, Jillian, Patricia, Christine, Casey, Catherine, Jordan, Renee, Kara, Natasha, Dana, Grace, Bianca, Madeline, Sabrina, Hailey, Julie, Deanna, Diana, Mariah, Kristin, Katlyn, Regina, Nina, Adriana, Cindy, Alexa, Kristina, Meghan, Destiny, Alana, Lydia, Elise, Holly, Heaven, Kiara, Angelique, Arlene, Cierra, Katelyn, Jessie, Karina, Alisha, Kassandra, Simone, Jasmin, Summer, Sandy, Juana, Lizbeth, Shanice, Candace, Marisol, Loren, Keisha, Kasey, Karla, Lacey, Makayla, Essence, Margarita, Ashleigh, Janice, Skylar, Sandra, Crystal, Susana, Alejandra, Makenna, Hanna, Tanya, Tyra, Britney, Marilyn, Dominique, Christy, Aliyah, Jazmine, Krista, Susie, Valeria, Arielle, Leticia, Rosemary, Latoya, Eileen, Marjorie, Corinne, Maricela, Araceli, Kailey, Destinee, Rebeca, Mariana, Janessa, Lorena, Michaela, Jocelyn, Adrienne, Marilyn, Lesley, Janie, Julianna, Janae,

Deja, Xiomara, Keely, Leila, Abbigail, Selina, Janelle, Katelin, Yazmin, Sonya, Dayana, Ashlee, Aubree, Kaylin, Annika, Lilly, Yesenia, Perla, Priscilla, Rocio, Tanisha, Cassidy, Alisa, Damaris, Christa, Rebekah, Graciela, Annabelle, Leanna, Allyson, Elsa, Janay, Kai, Ayla, Raquel, Belinda, Macie, Melina, Karlee, Tracey, Shayna, Karissa, Rosie, Reina, Elissa, Sonja, Lea, Precious, Keila, Jazmyn, Jaylene, Yasmine, Liliana, Kaylee, Isabela, Rosemarie, Estrella, Rhiannon, Karli, Kierra, Maricruz, Marisela, Guadalupe, Kiersten, Shelbie, Griselda, Kiera, Yuliana, Tia, Deasia, Anahi, Celia, Jasmyn, Corina, Anissa, Alondra, Kimber, Shayla, Cora, Aylin, Jolie, Kaiya, Jami, Marley, Laila, Ivana, Breanne, Kailee, Lilian, Isabel, Kaela, Ainsley, Yvette, Abigayle, Haylie, Laci, Tatyana, Taniya, Martina, Ashly, Alysia, Beatriz, Jaslyn, Kaelyn, Karly, Rylee, Corrine, Kierstin, Abagail, Amani, Silvia, Marcela, Esperanza, Jaden, Libby, Yadira, Nyla, Reanna, Aleah, Iliana, Nia, Shaniya, Dianna, Janiya, Aurora, Chaya, Dania, Danya, Luz, Micah, Naima, Reyna, Taniyah, Yajaira, Yoselin, Jalisa, Jazlyn, Taya, Tyla, Aliya, Anjali, Jaya, Shreya, Aniyah, Aniya, Cayla, Dariana, Galilea, Jania, Kimora, Ryann, Serenity, Shaylee, Shyanne, Tiara, Amira, Anaya, Anika, Cailyn, Calista, Elianna, Jaliyah, Kaila, Kamila, Kaylyn, Kylah, Samiya, Skyler, Yaretzi, Zaria, Dafne, Elisa, Elyse, Jaiden, Jayda, Kaya, Kayleen, Kelli, Khloe, Kinley, Lillie, Lyric, Makenzie, Malia, Nala, Nayeli, Raegan, Riya, Sanaa, Sanai, Sonia, Tania, Adelyn, Amara, Ayana, Brynlee, Elina, Jaylin, Kaitlin, Kenna, Kiana, Kianna, Leilani, Leyla, Mayra, Meadow, Nathalie, Nola, Samara, Yasmin, Zariah

Boys:
Michael, Christopher, Matthew, Joshua, Jacob, Nicholas, Andrew, Daniel, Tyler, Joseph, David, Brandon, Ryan, James, John, Zachary, Justin, William, Anthony, Jonathan, Robert, Kyle, Eric, Steven, Kevin, Thomas, Brian, Alexander, Cody, Benjamin, Adam, Aaron, Richard, Nathan, Patrick, Sean, Timothy, Caleb, Logan, Dustin, Jeremy, Austin

Natural Baby Names

Girls:
Willow, Jasmine, Lily, Daisy, Rose, Ivy, Hazel, Violet, Fern, Summer, Meadow, Laurel, Savannah, Aurora, Skye, Ocean, Ruby, Iris, Sierra, Autumn, Coral, Luna, Olive, Sage, Ember, Pearl, Sage, Clementine, Magnolia, Marigold, Rain, Breeze, Aurora, Willow, Ruby, Daisy, Rose, Laurel, Skye, Ocean, Iris, Sierra, Autumn, Luna, Sage, Ember, Pearl, Clementine, Marigold, Rain, Breeze

Boys:
River, Forrest, Canyon, Reed, Sky, Stone, Ocean, Aspen, Bear, Wolf, Cliff, Ridge, Brooks, Cedar, Fox, Hunter, Storm, Leaf, Rowan, Birch, Blaze, Ember, Orion, Forrest, Reed, Sky, Stone, Aspen, Bear, Wolf, Cliff, Ridge, Brooks, Cedar, Fox, Hunter, Storm, Leaf, Rowan, Birch, Blaze, Ember, Orion

Historical Figures Baby Names

Girls:
Eleanor, Cleopatra, Joan, Elizabeth, Marie, Catherine, Victoria, Anne, Mary, Florence, Rosa, Amelia, Harriet, Margaret, Jane, Eleanor, Elizabeth, Marie, Victoria, Anne, Mary, Florence, Rosa, Amelia, Harriet, Margaret, Jane

Boys:
Alexander, Julius, Napoleon, Abraham, Winston, Theodore, Martin, Leonardo, Isaac, Christopher, Galileo, Charles, Benjamin, Albert, Vincent, Nikola, Leonardo, Isaac, Christopher, Galileo, Charles, Benjamin, Albert, Vincent, Nikola

Ancient Roman Baby Names

Girls:
Julia, Flavia, Cornelia, Livia, Aurelia, Octavia, Claudia, Agrippina, Valeria, Minerva, Antonia, Tullia, Calpurnia, Lucretia, Drusilla, Julia, Flavia, Cornelia, Livia, Aurelia, Octavia, Claudia, Agrippina, Valeria, Minerva, Antonia, Tullia, Calpurnia, Lucretia, Drusilla

Boys:
Julius, Augustus, Marcus, Titus, Lucius, Cassius, Quintus, Octavius, Tiberius, Gaius, Cornelius, Octavian, Maximus, Marcellus, Julius, Augustus, Marcus, Titus, Lucius, Cassius, Quintus, Octavius, Tiberius, Gaius, Cornelius, Octavian, Maximus, Marcellus

Ancient Greek Baby Names

Girls:
Athena, Artemis, Persephone, Calliope, Cassandra, Daphne, Electra, Helen, Hera, Iris, Lysandra, Melaina, Naiad, Ophelia, Penelope, Thalia, Xanthe, Zoe, Althea, Cleo

Boys:
Apollo, Achilles, Alexander, Dionysus, Hector, Jason, Leonidas, Hermes, Perseus, Theseus, Atticus, Damon, Demetrius, Evander, Icarus, Lycurgus, Nicostratus, Odysseus, Pericles, Theron

Celebrity Baby Names

Girls:

Blue Ivy (Beyoncé and Jay-Z)
North (Kim Kardashian and Kanye West)
Apple (Gwyneth Paltrow and Chris Martin)
Suri (Tom Cruise and Katie Holmes)
Harper Seven (David and Victoria Beckham)
Rumi (Beyoncé and Jay-Z)
Bluebell Madonna (Geri Halliwell)
Luna Simone (John Legend and Chrissy Teigen)
Maxwell Drew (Jessica Simpson)
Dream (Rob Kardashian and Blac Chyna)
Birdie Mae (Jessica Simpson)
Atlas (Shay Mitchell)
Stormi (Kylie Jenner and Travis Scott)
Bodhi Soleil (Megan Fox and Brian Austin Green)
Marlowe (Sienna Miller)
Alba (Jessica Alba)
Willow (Pink and Carey Hart)
Coco (Courteney Cox and David Arquette)
Honor Marie (Jessica Alba)
Everly (Channing Tatum and Jenna Dewan)
Seraphina (Jennifer Garner and Ben Affleck)
Jagger (Ashlee Simpson and Evan Ross)
Rani (Kate Hudson)
True (Khloe Kardashian and Tristan Thompson)
Daisy Dove (Katy Perry and Orlando Bloom)
Sunday Rose (Nicole Kidman and Keith Urban)
Anja Louise (Alessandra Ambrosio)
Saylor (Kristin Cavallari and Jay Cutler)
Bryn (Bethenny Frankel)
Birdie Leigh (Busy Philipps)

Ella Bleu (John Travolta and Kelly Preston)
Jolie (Matt Damon)

Boys:

Saint (Kim Kardashian and Kanye West)
Reign (Kourtney Kardashian and Scott Disick)
Ace Knute (Jessica Simpson)
Pharaoh (Tyga and Blac Chyna)
Romeo (David and Victoria Beckham)
Maddox (Angelina Jolie and Brad Pitt)
Silas (Justin Timberlake and Jessica Biel)
Brooklyn (David and Victoria Beckham)
Rockwell Lloyd (Lucy Liu)
Memphis (Jason Aldean and Brittany Kerr)
Bronx Mowgli (Ashlee Simpson and Pete Wentz)
Romeo James (Rachel Zoe)
Moroccan (Mariah Carey and Nick Cannon)
Phoenix (Mel C)
Knox (Angelina Jolie and Brad Pitt)
Milan (Shakira and Gerard Piqué)
Zuma Nesta Rock (Gwen Stefani and Gavin Rossdale)
Jagger (Ashlee Simpson and Evan Ross)
Camden (Nick Lachey and Vanessa Minnillo)
Cruz (David and Victoria Beckham)
Apollo Bowie (Gwen Stefani and Gavin Rossdale)
Bear Blu (Alicia Silverstone)
Deacon (Reese Witherspoon and Ryan Phillippe)
Kingston (Gwen Stefani and Gavin Rossdale)
Max (Jennifer Lopez and Marc Anthony)
Samuel (Jennifer Garner and Ben Affleck)

Pagan Baby Names

Girls:

Luna - Meaning "moon", associated with feminine energy and intuition.

Willow - Symbolizing flexibility and resilience, often associated with nature and growth.

Gaia - Meaning "earth", symbolizing motherhood, fertility, and the nurturing aspect of nature.

Aurora - Derived from the Roman goddess of dawn, symbolizing new beginnings and enlightenment.

Freya - A Norse goddess associated with love, beauty, fertility, and war.

Morrigan - A Celtic goddess of war, fate, and death, embodying strength and power.

Selene - The Greek goddess of the moon, representing lunar magic, intuition, and mystery.

Brigid - An Irish goddess of healing, poetry, and smithcraft, symbolizing creativity and inspiration.

Persephone - The Greek goddess of spring and the underworld, symbolizing transformation and renewal.

Rowan - A tree with protective symbolism, often associated with strength, wisdom, and vision.

Rhiannon - A Welsh goddess associated with sovereignty, horses, and birds, symbolizing independence and strength.

Artemis - The Greek goddess of the hunt, wilderness, and childbirth, symbolizing independence and empowerment.

Isolde - Meaning "fair lady" or "beautiful", associated with love, passion, and tragic romance.

Cerridwen - A Welsh goddess of transformation, wisdom, and inspiration, symbolizing rebirth and magic.

Eris - The Greek goddess of chaos and strife, representing discord and the unexpected.

Hecate - A Greek goddess associated with witchcraft, magic, and the moon, symbolizing intuition and wisdom.

Maeve - Meaning "she who intoxicates", associated with sovereignty, femininity, and sensuality.

Arianrhod - A Welsh goddess associated with the moon, fertility, and fate, symbolizing cosmic cycles and transformation.

Morgana - Derived from the Welsh name for the sorceress Morgan le Fay, symbolizing mystery and enchantment.

Thalia - From Greek mythology, one of the nine Muses, representing comedy and idyllic poetry.

Anthea - Meaning "flower", symbolizing beauty, grace, and the blossoming of life.

Elara - A moon of Jupiter named after a lover of Zeus, symbolizing devotion and endurance.

Nyx - The Greek goddess of the night, symbolizing darkness, mystery, and the unseen.

Ondine - A water nymph from European folklore, symbolizing beauty, grace, and fluidity.

Tanith - A Phoenician lunar goddess associated with fertility, love, and the cycle of life.

Astra - Meaning "star", symbolizing guidance, hope, and the celestial realm.

Epona - A Celtic goddess associated with horses, fertility, and abundance, symbolizing freedom and strength.

Fawn - Symbolizing innocence, gentleness, and the natural world.

Hestia - The Greek goddess of hearth and home, representing warmth, hospitality, and domestic harmony.

Lilith - A figure from Jewish folklore, symbolizing independence, sexuality, and feminine power.

Niamh - Meaning "brightness" or "radiance", symbolizing beauty, vitality, and joy.

Phoebe - The Greek Titaness of the moon, associated with prophecy, wisdom, and illumination.

Seraphina - Derived from "seraphim", the highest order of angels, symbolizing divine love and purity.

Thalia - Meaning "blooming", symbolizing youth, beauty, and the flourishing of life.

Boys:

Odin - The chief god in Norse mythology, associated with wisdom, knowledge, and warfare.

Thor - The Norse god of thunder, symbolizing strength, protection, and courage.

Apollo - The Greek god of music, poetry, prophecy, and healing, symbolizing creativity and harmony.

Loki - A complex figure in Norse mythology, symbolizing mischief, trickery, and transformation.

Orion - A hunter in Greek mythology, symbolizing strength, bravery, and the pursuit of excellence.

Freyr - The Norse god of fertility, prosperity, and peace, symbolizing abundance and joy.

Cernunnos - A Celtic god associated with nature, fertility, and the cycle of life, symbolizing wildness and vitality.

Pan - The Greek god of nature, shepherds, and rustic music, symbolizing wilderness and primal instincts.

Ares - The Greek god of war, representing strength, courage, and conflict.

Finn - Meaning "fair" or "white", symbolizing purity, clarity, and wisdom.

Apollo - The Greek god of music, poetry, prophecy, and healing, symbolizing creativity and harmony.

Bran - A figure from Welsh mythology associated with protection, prophecy, and wisdom.

Dagda - The chief god in Irish mythology, symbolizing strength, abundance, and wisdom.

Hermes - The Greek god

Shakespeare Names

Girls:

Juliet - From Shakespeare's "Romeo and Juliet", symbolizing love, passion, and tragedy.

Ophelia - From "Hamlet", symbolizing innocence, madness, and tragic fate.

Rosalind - From "As You Like It", symbolizing wit, intelligence, and independence.

Cordelia - From "King Lear", symbolizing loyalty, honesty, and strength.

Viola - From "Twelfth Night", symbolizing disguise, identity, and love.

Portia - From "The Merchant of Venice", symbolizing intelligence, courage, and justice.

Desdemona - From "Othello", symbolizing innocence, love, and tragedy.

Beatrice - From "Much Ado About Nothing", symbolizing wit, humor, and independence.

Helena - From "A Midsummer Night's Dream", symbolizing unrequited love, perseverance, and transformation.

Bianca - From "Othello", symbolizing innocence, jealousy, and manipulation.

Miranda - From "The Tempest", symbolizing innocence, wonder, and discovery.

Hero - From "Much Ado About Nothing", symbolizing purity, love, and deception.

Isabella - From "Measure for Measure", symbolizing virtue, integrity, and moral strength.

Nerissa - From "The Merchant of Venice", symbolizing loyalty, intelligence, and resourcefulness.

Imogen - From "Cymbeline", symbolizing strength, resilience, and forgiveness.

Titania - From "A Midsummer Night's Dream", symbolizing power, beauty, and enchantment.

Boys:

Romeo - From "Romeo and Juliet", symbolizing love, passion, and romanticism.

Hamlet - From "Hamlet", symbolizing indecision, madness, and tragic fate.

Oberon - From "A Midsummer Night's Dream", symbolizing power, manipulation, and magic.

Macbeth - From "Macbeth", symbolizing ambition, guilt, and corruption.

Prospero - From "The Tempest", symbolizing wisdom, power, and forgiveness.

Antonio - From "The Merchant of Venice", symbolizing friendship, loyalty, and sacrifice.

Orlando - From "As You Like It", symbolizing love, bravery, and transformation.

Tybalt - From "Romeo and Juliet", symbolizing aggression, rivalry, and tragedy.

Sebastian - From "Twelfth Night", symbolizing loyalty, adventure, and identity.

Laertes - From "Hamlet", symbolizing honor, revenge, and family loyalty.

Cassio - From "Othello", symbolizing integrity, friendship, and manipulation.

Ferdinand - From "The Tempest", symbolizing love, innocence, and romanticism.

Mercutio - From "Romeo and Juliet", symbolizing wit, humor, and tragedy.

Petruchio - From "The Taming of the Shrew", symbolizing wit, dominance, and transformation.

Malvolio - From "Twelfth Night", symbolizing pride, arrogance, and humiliation.

Horatio - From "Hamlet", symbolizing loyalty, friendship, and integrity.

Paris - From "Romeo and Juliet", symbolizing love, rivalry, and tragedy.

Astrological Names

Aries - The Ram, representing determination and leadership.

Taurus - The Bull, symbolizing strength and stability.

Gemini - The Twins, signifying duality and adaptability.

Cancer - The Crab, symbolizing sensitivity and protection.

Leo - The Lion, representing courage and loyalty.

Virgo - The Virgin, symbolizing practicality and attention to detail.

Libra - The Scales, representing balance and harmony.

Scorpio - The Scorpion, symbolizing intensity and transformation.

Sagittarius - The Archer, representing adventure and optimism.

Capricorn - The Sea-Goat, symbolizing ambition and resilience.

Aquarius - The Water-Bearer, representing innovation and independence.

Pisces - The Fish, symbolizing compassion and intuition.

Luna - Derived from the Latin word for "moon," symbolizing femininity and intuition.

Sol - Latin for "sun," symbolizing vitality and warmth.

Stella - Latin for "star," symbolizing brightness and guidance.

Celeste - From Latin origin meaning "heavenly," symbolizing purity and divinity.

Orion - Named after the constellation, symbolizing strength and resilience.

Venus - Named after the Roman goddess of love and beauty.

Mars - Named after the Roman god of war, symbolizing strength and courage.

Jupiter - Named after the Roman king of the gods, symbolizing expansion and abundance.

Saturn - Named after the Roman god of agriculture, symbolizing discipline and responsibility.

Neptune - Named after the Roman god of the sea, symbolizing mystery and spirituality.

Pluto - Named after the Roman god of the underworld, symbolizing transformation and rebirth.

Mercury - Named after the Roman messenger god, symbolizing communication and intellect.

Uranus - Named after the Greek god of the sky, symbolizing innovation and revolution.

Nova - Latin for "new," symbolizing fresh beginnings and transformation.

Phoenix - Symbolizing rebirth and regeneration, derived from Greek mythology.

Cassiopeia - Named after the queen in Greek mythology, symbolizing beauty and pride.

Andromeda - Named after the princess in Greek mythology, symbolizing courage and sacrifice.

Sirius - The brightest star in the sky, symbolizing guidance and clarity.

Vega - Named after the brightest star in the constellation Lyra, symbolizing strength and brilliance.

Altair - Named after the brightest star in the constellation Aquila, symbolizing ambition and achievement.

Aldebaran - The brightest star in the Taurus constellation, symbolizing determination and endurance.

Antares - The brightest star in the Scorpius constellation, symbolizing intensity and passion.

Bellatrix - Latin for "female warrior," symbolizing strength and resilience.

Betelgeuse - Named after a red supergiant star, symbolizing power and vitality.

Lyra - Named after the lyre of Orpheus in Greek mythology, symbolizing creativity and expression.

Draco - Latin for "dragon," symbolizing mystery and strength.

Cetus - Named after the sea monster in Greek mythology, symbolizing power and depth.

Corona - Latin for "crown," symbolizing authority and nobility.

Electra - Named after one of the seven sisters in Greek mythology, symbolizing beauty and grace.

Eos - Greek goddess of the dawn, symbolizing new beginnings and hope.

Helios - Greek god of the sun, symbolizing vitality and energy.

Hyperion - One of the Titans in Greek mythology, symbolizing wisdom and enlightenment.

Lysander - Greek name meaning "liberator," symbolizing freedom and independence.

Miranda - Latin for "admirable," symbolizing grace and elegance.

Oberon - King of the fairies in Shakespeare's "A Midsummer Night's Dream," symbolizing magic and mystery.

Pallas - Named after the Greek goddess of wisdom, symbolizing intellect and strategy.

Pandora - From Greek mythology, symbolizing curiosity and discovery.

Persephone - Greek goddess of spring and queen of the underworld, symbolizing transformation and renewal.

Geographic Names

Aspen - Named after the tree known for its resilience, symbolizing strength and endurance.

Brooklyn - Derived from the Dutch name meaning "broken land," symbolizing resilience and adaptability.

Dakota - Native American name meaning "ally" or "friend," symbolizing companionship and loyalty.

Florence - Derived from the Latin name meaning "flourishing" or "prosperous," symbolizing growth and abundance.

Georgia - Derived from the Greek name meaning "farmer" or "earthworker," symbolizing connection to the land and fertility.

Hudson - English surname derived from Old English meaning "son of Hudde," symbolizing lineage and heritage.

India - Named after the country, symbolizing diversity and cultural richness.

Jordan - Derived from the Hebrew name meaning "to descend" or "flow down," symbolizing purification and renewal.

Kenya - Named after the African country, symbolizing beauty and wilderness.

London - Named after the capital city of England, symbolizing tradition and modernity.

Milan - Named after the city in Italy, symbolizing elegance and sophistication.

Paris - Named after the capital city of France, symbolizing romance and beauty.

Phoenix - Symbolizing rebirth and renewal, derived from the mythical bird that rises from its own ashes.

Sydney - Named after the city in Australia, symbolizing vitality and energy.

Vienna - Named after the capital city of Austria, symbolizing culture and refinement.

Adelaide - Derived from the Germanic name meaning "noble" or "nobility," symbolizing grace and dignity.

Cairo - Named after the capital city of Egypt, symbolizing history and civilization.

Dallas - Derived from the Scottish surname meaning "meadow dwelling," symbolizing tranquility and nature.

Everest - Named after the highest mountain in the world, symbolizing strength and aspiration.

Havana - Named after the capital city of Cuba, symbolizing vibrancy and energy.

Kingston - Derived from the English surname meaning "king's town," symbolizing royalty and leadership.

Lisbon - Named after the capital city of Portugal, symbolizing exploration and discovery.

Madison - Derived from the English surname meaning "son of Maud," symbolizing strength and independence.

Oslo - Named after the capital city of Norway, symbolizing peace and tranquility.

Sahara - Named after the desert in North Africa, symbolizing endurance and resilience.

Valencia - Named after the city in Spain, symbolizing strength and vitality.

Zurich - Named after the city in Switzerland, symbolizing prosperity and stability.

Geneva - Named after the city in Switzerland, symbolizing peace and harmony.

Houston - Named after the city in Texas, symbolizing resilience and determination.

Lima - Named after the capital city of Peru, symbolizing history and culture.

Manila - Named after the capital city of the Philippines, symbolizing diversity and resilience.

Panama - Named after the country, symbolizing connection and unity.

Rio - Named after the city in Brazil, symbolizing energy and vitality.

Santiago - Named after the capital city of Chile, symbolizing strength and resilience.

Tahoe - Named after Lake Tahoe, symbolizing serenity and tranquility.

Vegas - Named after the city in Nevada, symbolizing excitement and entertainment.

Austin - Named after the capital city of Texas, symbolizing strength and determination.

Caspian - Named after the Caspian Sea, symbolizing depth and mystery.

Denver - Named after the city in Colorado, symbolizing ruggedness and resilience.

Gender Neutral Names

Avery - Of Old English origin, meaning "ruler of the elves," symbolizing leadership and mystical connection.

Riley - Of Irish origin, meaning "courageous" or "valiant," symbolizing bravery and strength.

Jordan - Derived from the Hebrew name meaning "to descend" or "flow down," symbolizing purification and renewal.

Quinn - Of Irish origin, meaning "wise" or "counsel," symbolizing intelligence and guidance.

Cameron - Of Scottish origin, meaning "crooked nose" or "bent nose," symbolizing uniqueness and individuality.

Dakota - Native American name meaning "ally" or "friend," symbolizing companionship and loyalty.

Morgan - Of Welsh origin, meaning "sea-born" or "sea chief," symbolizing strength and adaptability.

Taylor - Of English origin, meaning "cutter of cloth" or "to tailor," symbolizing craftsmanship and precision.

Casey - Of Irish origin, meaning "vigilant" or "watchful," symbolizing awareness and intuition.

Jamie - Of Hebrew origin, meaning "supplanter" or "one who follows," symbolizing adaptability and persistence.

Emerson - Of English origin, meaning "son of Emery" or "industrious leader," symbolizing productivity and leadership.

Payton - Of English origin, meaning "fighter's estate" or "warrior's town," symbolizing resilience and strength.

Sydney - Of English origin, meaning "wide island" or "wide meadow," symbolizing openness and expansiveness.

Alexis - Of Greek origin, meaning "defender" or "helper," symbolizing protection and support.

Harper - Derived from the Old English word for "harp player," symbolizing creativity and expression.

Hayden - Of English origin, meaning "valley with hay" or "hay hill," symbolizing nourishment and growth.

Rowan - Named after the rowan tree, symbolizing protection and intuition.

Finley - Of Scottish origin, meaning "fair-haired hero" or "fair warrior," symbolizing courage and fairness.

Reese - Of Welsh origin, meaning "enthusiastic" or "ardent," symbolizing passion and energy.

Sage - Referring to the aromatic herb, symbolizing wisdom and clarity.

Ancient Irish Names

Aedan - "Little fire," symbolizing passion and energy.

Ailbhe - "White," symbolizing purity and innocence.

Aine - "Radiance" or "splendor," symbolizing beauty and brightness.

Bairrfhionn - "Fair-haired," symbolizing light and clarity.

Beibhinn - "Fair lady," symbolizing grace and elegance.

Bran - "Raven," symbolizing intelligence and cunning.

Brigid - From the Celtic goddess of fire, poetry, and wisdom.

Caoimhe - "Gentle," symbolizing kindness and compassion.

Cian - "Ancient" or "enduring," symbolizing strength and resilience.

Clodagh - From the name of a river in County Tipperary, symbolizing flow and movement.

Colm - "Dove," symbolizing peace and harmony.

Cormac - "Charioteer," symbolizing skill and leadership.

Deirdre - "Sorrowful" or "broken-hearted," symbolizing resilience and emotional depth.

Eimear - "Swift" or "nimble," symbolizing agility and quick thinking.

Eoin - "God is gracious," symbolizing divine favor.

Faolan - "Little wolf," symbolizing loyalty and fierceness.

Fionnuala - "Fair shoulder," symbolizing grace and beauty.

Grainne - "Grain" or "kernel," symbolizing abundance and fertility.

Iarlaith - "Earl" or "nobleman," symbolizing aristocracy and honor.

Laoise - "Radiant girl," symbolizing brightness and warmth.

Liadan - "Grey lady," symbolizing wisdom and maturity.

Maeve - "Intoxicating," symbolizing allure and charm.

Niamh - "Bright" or "radiant," symbolizing beauty and vitality.

Oisin - "Little deer," symbolizing grace and agility.

Oran - "Song" or "poem," symbolizing creativity and expression.

Riona - "Queenly," symbolizing leadership and authority.

Ronan - "Little seal," symbolizing curiosity and playfulness.

Saoirse - "Freedom" or "liberty," symbolizing independence and autonomy.

Senan - "Wise old man," symbolizing wisdom and experience.

Sinead - Derived from "Jeanette," symbolizing grace and elegance.

Sorcha - "Bright" or "radiant," symbolizing warmth and vitality.

Tadhg - "Poet" or "philosopher," symbolizing creativity and insight.

Aoife - "Beautiful" or "radiant," symbolizing elegance and charm.

Art - "Bear," symbolizing strength and courage.

Blathnaid - "Flower" or "blossom," symbolizing beauty and growth.

Cathal - "Mighty in battle," symbolizing strength and bravery.

Ciara - "Dark-haired" or "dark beauty," symbolizing mystery and allure.

Cliona - "Shapely" or "well-proportioned," symbolizing beauty and grace.

Colleen - Derived from the Irish word for "girl," symbolizing youth and innocence.

Conor - "Lover of hounds," symbolizing loyalty and companionship.

Darragh - "Oak tree," symbolizing strength and endurance.

Eilis - Derived from "Elizabeth," symbolizing consecration and dedication.

Enda - "Bird-like" or "swift," symbolizing agility and freedom.

Eoghan - "Born of the yew tree," symbolizing longevity and resilience.

Fergus - "Man of vigor," symbolizing strength and vitality.

Fiona - "Fair" or "white," symbolizing purity and innocence.

Gearoid - "Spear carrier," symbolizing bravery and valor.

Grania - Variant of "Grainne," symbolizing abundance and fertility.

Lir - "Sea" or "ocean," symbolizing depth and mystery.

Lorcan - "Little fierce one," symbolizing determination and courage.

Mairead - Derived from "Margaret," symbolizing pearl-like beauty.

Muireann - "Sea white," symbolizing purity and clarity.

Niall - "Champion" or "passionate," symbolizing victory and fervor.

Orla - "Golden princess," symbolizing royalty and beauty.

Padraig - "Noble" or "illustrious," symbolizing honor and dignity.

Roisin - "Little rose," symbolizing beauty and delicacy.

Sean - "God is gracious," symbolizing divine favor and blessing.

Siobhan - Derived from "Joan," symbolizing God's gift of grace.

Turlough - "From the land of the lakes," symbolizing tranquility and serenity.

Aisling - "Dream" or "vision," symbolizing inspiration and imagination.

Artur - Derived from "Arthur," symbolizing strength and leadership.

Bevan - "Young soldier," symbolizing courage and bravery.

Branwen - "Blessed raven," symbolizing divine favor and wisdom.

Briana - Derived from "Brian," symbolizing strength and nobility.

Ciaran - "Little dark one," symbolizing mystery and allure.

Colla - "Young warrior," symbolizing bravery and courage.

Conall - "Strong wolf," symbolizing strength and ferocity.

Donal - "World ruler," symbolizing authority and leadership.

Eanna - "Bird-like" or "swift," symbolizing freedom and agility.

Eileen - Derived from "Helen," symbolizing light and clarity.

Eireann - "Ireland," symbolizing patriotism and heritage.

Evin - "Young warrior," symbolizing courage and strength.

Fia - "Wild deer," symbolizing freedom and grace.

Fionn - "Fair" or "blond," symbolizing purity and clarity.

Gobnait - "Smith" or "blacksmith," symbolizing craftsmanship and skill.

Lughaidh - "Light" or "brightness," symbolizing illumination and enlightenment.

Malachy - "Follower of Saint Columba," symbolizing faith and devotion.

Morna - "Affection" or "beloved," symbolizing love and tenderness.

Murtagh - "Sea warrior," symbolizing strength and resilience.

Nessa - "Not gentle" or "not soft," symbolizing strength and determination.

Orna - "Sallow" or "pale green," symbolizing growth and renewal.

Sadhbh - "Sweet" or "gentle," symbolizing kindness and tenderness.

Ancient Scottish Names

Sheena - Scottish form of Jane, symbolizing God's gift of grace.

Skye - Named after the Scottish island, symbolizing vastness and freedom.

Stewart - Derived from the Old English word for "steward" or "keeper of the estate," symbolizing responsibility and care.

Struan - Derived from the Gaelic word for "stream," symbolizing flow and movement.

Sutherland - Named after the Scottish county, symbolizing heritage and lineage.

Tavish - Scottish form of Thomas, meaning "twin," symbolizing companionship and duality.

Torquil - "Thor's kettle" or "Thor's cauldron," symbolizing strength and power.

Urquhart - Derived from the Gaelic word for "by the thicket," symbolizing nature and wilderness.

Wallace - Derived from the Old English word for "foreigner" or "Welshman," symbolizing diversity and cultural richness.

Yarrow - Named after the Scottish river, symbolizing flow and adaptability.

Ailpein - Scottish form of Alpin, meaning "white," symbolizing purity and innocence.

Ainslie - Variant of Ainsley, symbolizing openness and growth.

Airell - Possibly derived from the Gaelic word for "nobleman," symbolizing honor and dignity.

Allister - Variant of Alistair, symbolizing strength and leadership.

Angusina - Feminine form of Angus, symbolizing individuality and resilience.

Annag - Diminutive of Annabel, symbolizing transition and journey.

Archibald - "Genuine" or "bold," symbolizing authenticity and courage.

Artair - Scottish form of Arthur, meaning "bear," symbolizing strength and courage.

Baird - Derived from the Scottish word for "minstrel" or "poet," symbolizing creativity and expression.

Barclay - Derived from the Scottish surname meaning "birch tree clearing," symbolizing growth and renewal.

Blaine - Derived from the Gaelic word for "yellow," symbolizing brightness and clarity.

Blaire - Variant of Blair, symbolizing openness and expansiveness.

Blythe - Derived from the Old English word for "joyous" or "carefree," symbolizing happiness and freedom.

Bonny - Derived from the Scottish word for "beautiful" or "attractive," symbolizing charm and attractiveness.

Braeden - Variant of Braden, meaning "broad valley," symbolizing openness and expansiveness.

Branan - Possibly derived from the Gaelic word for "raven," symbolizing intelligence and cunning.

Breac - Derived from the Gaelic word for "speckled" or "variegated," symbolizing diversity and uniqueness.

Bree - Derived from the Scottish word for "hill," symbolizing elevation and perspective.

Breena - Feminine form of Breen, symbolizing strength and resilience.

Briar - Derived from the Scottish word for "thorny patch," symbolizing protection and defense.

Brice - Derived from the Gaelic word for "speckled" or "freckled," symbolizing uniqueness and individuality.

Bryce - Variant of Brice, symbolizing uniqueness and individuality.

Caden - Derived from the Gaelic word for "spirit of battle," symbolizing strength and determination.

Cailin - Derived from the Scottish word for "girl" or "lass," symbolizing youth and innocence.

Cailyn - Variant of Cailin, symbolizing youth and innocence.

Cairbre - Possibly derived from the Gaelic word for "charioteer," symbolizing skill and leadership.

Calum - Variant of Callum, symbolizing peace and harmony.

Carmichael - Derived from the Gaelic word for "son of Michael," symbolizing divine protection.

Cassidy - Derived from the Scottish surname meaning "curly-haired," symbolizing uniqueness and individuality.

Chisholm - Derived from the Gaelic word for "hazel wood," symbolizing wisdom and intuition.

Clark - Derived from the Scottish word for "scribe" or "clerk," symbolizing knowledge and literacy.

Collin - Derived from the Scottish word for "young creature," symbolizing youth and vitality.

Connall - Variant of Conall, meaning "strong wolf," symbolizing strength and ferocity.

Craig - Derived from the Scottish word for "rock" or "crag," symbolizing stability and endurance.

Craigie - Diminutive of Craig, symbolizing stability and endurance.

Dallas - Derived from the Scottish surname meaning "from the dales," symbolizing connection to nature.

Duff - Derived from the Gaelic word for "dark" or "black," symbolizing mystery and depth.

Duncan - "Brown warrior" or "dark warrior," symbolizing strength and resilience.

Dunstan - Derived from the Gaelic word for "brown stone," symbolizing solidity and stability.

Eairdsidh - Scottish form of Archie, meaning "genuine" or "bold," symbolizing authenticity and courage.

Ancient English Names

Earnest - Derived from Old English elements meaning "serious" or "sincere," symbolizing honesty and authenticity.

Ecgberht - Old English name meaning "bright edge," symbolizing sharpness and clarity.

Edric - Old English name meaning "wealthy ruler," symbolizing prosperity and leadership.

Edwin - Old English name meaning "rich friend," symbolizing abundance and companionship.

Eldred - Old English name meaning "old counsel," symbolizing wisdom and experience.

Elfwin - Old English name meaning "elf friend," symbolizing harmony with nature.

Ethelbert - Old English name meaning "noble bright," symbolizing honor and brilliance.

Ethelred - Old English name meaning "noble counsel," symbolizing wisdom and leadership.

Godric - Old English name meaning "godly ruler," symbolizing divine authority.

Godwin - Old English name meaning "friend of god," symbolizing divine favor.

Guthrie - Old English name meaning "war leader," symbolizing strength and valor.

Leofric - Old English name meaning "dear ruler," symbolizing beloved leadership.

Leofwin - Old English name meaning "dear friend," symbolizing cherished companionship.

Oswin - Old English name meaning "godly friend," symbolizing divine companionship.

Radulf - Old English name meaning "counsel of the wolf," symbolizing wisdom and cunning.

Seaward - Old English name meaning "sea guardian," symbolizing protection over the waters.

Siward - Old English name meaning "victory guardian," symbolizing triumph and protection.

Thurstan - Old English name meaning "Thor's stone," symbolizing strength and resilience.

Walford - Old English name meaning "river crossing of the Welsh," symbolizing cultural intersection.

Wulfric - Old English name meaning "wolf power," symbolizing strength and ferocity.

Wynstan - Old English name meaning "joy stone," symbolizing happiness and stability.

Ancient Latin Names

Aemilianus - Latin name derived from "Aemilius," meaning "rival."

Agrippina - Feminine form of "Agrippinus," meaning "born feet first" or "wild horse."

Albinus - Latin name derived from "Albus," meaning "white" or "bright."

Antonius - Latin form of "Anthony," possibly meaning "priceless" or "of inestimable worth."

Apollonius - Latinized form of the Greek name "Apollonios," meaning "belonging to Apollo."

Augustus - Latin name derived from "augere," meaning "to increase" or "to augment."

Aurelius - Latin name derived from "Aureus," meaning "golden" or "gilded."

Cassius - Roman family name possibly derived from Latin "cassus," meaning "empty" or "vain."

Cincinnatus - Roman family name derived from Latin "cincinnus," meaning "curly-haired."

Claudius - Roman family name possibly derived from Latin "claudus," meaning "lame" or "limping."

Cornelia - Feminine form of "Cornelius," possibly derived from "cornu," meaning "horn."

Decimus - Latin name meaning "tenth," often used as a praenomen (given name).

Drusus - Roman family name, possibly derived from the Celtic elements meaning "strong" or "sturdy."

Fabius - Roman family name derived from Latin "faba," meaning "bean."

Flavius - Roman family name derived from Latin "flavus," meaning "yellow" or "blond."

Gaius - Ancient Roman praenomen (given name) of uncertain meaning.

Julius - Roman family name, possibly derived from Greek "ioulos," meaning "downy-bearded" or "youthful."

Junius - Roman family name, possibly derived from Latin "iuniores," meaning "young ones."

Lavinia - Feminine form of "Lavinus," possibly meaning "purity" or "clear."

Lucius - Roman praenomen (given name) derived from Latin "lux," meaning "light."

Marcellus - Roman family name, a diminutive of "Marcus," possibly meaning "hammer" or "warlike."

Maximus - Latin name meaning "greatest" or "largest."

Octavius - Latin name derived from "octavus," meaning "eighth."

Pomponius - Roman family name derived from Latin "pompa," meaning "procession" or "parade."

Priscilla - Feminine form of "Priscus," meaning "ancient" or "venerable."

Quintus - Latin name meaning "fifth," often used as a praenomen.

Regulus - Latin name meaning "little king" or "prince."

Sextus - Latin name meaning "sixth," often used as a praenomen.

Tiberius - Roman praenomen derived from "Tiberis," the river Tiber.

Ancient Hebrew Names

Abigail - Means "my father is joy," symbolizing happiness and familial connection.

Abraham - Means "father of many" or "father of a multitude," symbolizing paternal leadership.

Adam - Means "man" or "earth," symbolizing humanity and earthly origins.

Benjamin - Means "son of the right hand," symbolizing favor and strength.

Caleb - Means "faithful" or "loyal," symbolizing trustworthiness and devotion.

Daniel - Means "God is my judge," symbolizing divine justice and wisdom.

Deborah - Means "bee," symbolizing industry and community.

Elijah - Means "my God is Yahweh," symbolizing devotion and faithfulness.

Esther - Possibly means "star," symbolizing beauty and guidance.

Ezekiel - Means "God will strengthen," symbolizing divine support and empowerment.

Isaac - Means "he will laugh," symbolizing joy and laughter.

Isaiah - Means "Yahweh is salvation," symbolizing divine deliverance.

Jacob - Means "supplanter" or "holder of the heel," symbolizing cunning and perseverance.

Joshua - Means "Yahweh is salvation," symbolizing divine assistance and guidance.

Leah - Possibly means "weary" or "tired," symbolizing endurance and strength.

Miriam - Possibly means "sea of bitterness" or "sea of sorrow," symbolizing resilience and depth.

Moses - Possibly means "drawn out" or "taken from water," symbolizing divine rescue and guidance.

Naomi - Means "pleasantness" or "sweetness," symbolizing kindness and amiability.

Nathan - Means "he gave" or "gift of God," symbolizing divine favor and generosity.

Rachel - Means "ewe" or "female sheep," symbolizing gentleness and nurturing.

Ruth - Means "friend" or "companion," symbolizing loyalty and companionship.

Samuel - Means "heard by God" or "name of God," symbolizing divine communication and connection.

Sarah - Means "princess" or "noblewoman," symbolizing royalty and dignity.

Solomon - Means "peaceful" or "peace-loving," symbolizing tranquility and wisdom.

Zechariah - Means "Yahweh remembers," symbolizing divine memory and faithfulness.

Ancient Arabic Names

Aisha - Means "alive" or "living," symbolizing vitality and energy.

Ali - Means "noble" or "sublime," symbolizing honor and dignity.

Amira - Means "princess" or "commander," symbolizing royalty and leadership.

Bilal - Means "moist" or "refreshing," symbolizing vitality and rejuvenation.

Fatima - Means "captivating" or "chaste," symbolizing purity and allure.

Hamza - Means "strong" or "steadfast," symbolizing resilience and fortitude.

Hassan - Means "handsome" or "good," symbolizing beauty and virtue.

Khadija - Means "premature" or "premature child," symbolizing early arrival and importance.

Layla - Means "night" or "dark beauty," symbolizing mystery and allure.

Malik - Means "king" or "master," symbolizing sovereignty and authority.

Mariam - Arabic form of "Mary," possibly meaning "beloved" or "wished-for child," symbolizing affection and desire.

Muhammad - Means "praised" or "praiseworthy," symbolizing commendation and honor.

Nour - Means "light" or "illumination," symbolizing enlightenment and clarity.

Omar - Means "flourishing" or "prosperous," symbolizing growth and success.

Rania - Means "gazing" or "looking at," symbolizing observation and awareness.

Salim - Means "safe" or "sound," symbolizing security and protection.

Samira - Means "companion in evening talk" or "friend of the night," symbolizing camaraderie and friendship.

Talal - Means "nice" or "gentle," symbolizing kindness and tenderness.

Yasmin - Means "jasmine flower," symbolizing grace and delicacy.

Zainab - Means "fragrant flower" or "beauty," symbolizing elegance and charm.

Ancient Eqyptian Names

Ra - Sun god
Nefertari - Beautiful companion
Tutankhamun - Living image of Amun
Cleopatra - Glory of the father
Akhenaten - Effective for Aten
Hatshepsut - Foremost of noblewomen
Thutmose - Born of Thoth
Nefertiti - The beautiful one has come
Amenhotep - Amun is satisfied
Senenmut - Mother's brother
Ankhesenamun - She lives for Amun
Khufu - Protected by Khnum
Seti - Man of Set
Sobekneferu - Beauty of Sobek
Amenemhat - Amun is foremost
Meritaten - Beloved of Aten
Ramses - Born of Ra
Neferneferuaten - Beautiful are the beauties of Aten
Ankhtifi - Living image of Anubis
Nefertem - Beautiful one who closes or shuts
Ptahhotep - Ptah is pleased
Sobekhotep - Sobek is satisfied
Merit - Beloved
Neferkare - Beautiful is the ka of Ra
Mentuhotep - Montu is satisfied
Merneptah - Beloved of Ptah
Akhenre - Effective for Ra
Sobekemsaf - Sobek is his protection
Amunhotep - Amun is satisfied
Tuthmosis - Born of Thoth
Nefer - Beautiful
Khafre - Appearing like Ra
Sobek - Crocodile god
Khepri - Morning sun god

Tawaret - Goddess of childbirth and fertility
Maatkare - Truth is the ka of Ra
Ahmose - Born of the moon god
Horemheb - Horus is in jubilation
Hatshepsut - Foremost of noblewomen
Ankhesenpaaten - She lives for Aten
Senusret - Man of goddess Wosret
Tetisheri - The wife of the falcon
Khaemwaset - He appears in Thebes

Royal Names

Alexander - Meaning "defender of the people," symbolizing protection and support.

Victoria - Meaning "victory," symbolizing triumph and success.

Edward - Meaning "wealthy guardian," symbolizing prosperity and protection.

Elizabeth - Meaning "pledged to God," symbolizing devotion and commitment.

William - Meaning "resolute protector," symbolizing strength and guardianship.

Catherine - Meaning "pure," symbolizing innocence and clarity.

Henry - Meaning "ruler of the household," symbolizing leadership and authority.

Margaret - Meaning "pearl," symbolizing beauty and preciousness.

Richard - Meaning "brave power," symbolizing courage and strength.

Eleanor - Meaning "bright, shining one," symbolizing radiance and brilliance.

Charles - Meaning "free man," symbolizing independence and liberty.

Mary - Meaning "beloved," symbolizing affection and endearment.

Philip - Meaning "lover of horses," symbolizing nobility and elegance.

Matilda - Meaning "battle-mighty," symbolizing strength and valor.

Arthur - Meaning "bear," symbolizing courage and resilience.

Alexandra - Feminine form of Alexander, symbolizing protection and support.

Frederick - Meaning "peaceful ruler," symbolizing harmony and leadership.

Adelaide - Meaning "noble type," symbolizing aristocracy and dignity.

George - Meaning "farmer," symbolizing diligence and hard work.

Anne - Meaning "grace," symbolizing elegance and charm.

Louis - Meaning "renowned warrior," symbolizing fame and valor.

Leopold - Meaning "bold people," symbolizing courage and bravery.

Edmund - Meaning "rich protector," symbolizing wealth and defense.

Charlotte - Meaning "free man," symbolizing independence and liberty.

Nautical Names

Marina - Meaning "of the sea," symbolizing a connection to the ocean.

Oceanus - Named after the Greek god of the ocean, symbolizing vastness and power.

Ariel - Meaning "lion of God," associated with the spirit of the air and the sea.

Pearl - Symbolizing beauty and purity, reminiscent of treasures found in the ocean.

Triton - Named after the Greek god of the sea, symbolizing strength and authority.

Marlin - Inspired by the large and powerful ocean fish, symbolizing determination and endurance.

Nereus - Named after the ancient Greek sea god, symbolizing the wisdom of the sea.

Coral - Symbolizing delicate beauty and the vibrant life found in coral reefs.

Seabrook - Meaning "near the brook by the sea," evoking coastal imagery.

Mira - Meaning "sea" in Latin, symbolizing a connection to the ocean.

Kai - Hawaiian name meaning "sea," symbolizing a deep affinity for the ocean.

Cove - Evoking images of sheltered coastal areas, symbolizing tranquility and protection.

Finn - Meaning "fair" or "white," reminiscent of ocean foam and waves.

Coralie - Diminutive of Coral, symbolizing the delicate and colorful life of coral reefs.

Drake - Inspired by the sea-faring explorer Sir Francis Drake, symbolizing adventure and discovery.

Calypso - Named after the sea nymph in Greek mythology, symbolizing mystery and allure.

Hudson - Meaning "son of the sea," evoking maritime imagery and exploration.

Lagoon - Symbolizing serene and shallow coastal waters, often associated with tropical paradises.

Neptune - Named after the Roman god of the sea, symbolizing power and majesty.

Sandy - Evoking images of sandy beaches and coastal landscapes, symbolizing warmth and relaxation.

Wave - Symbolizing the rhythmic motion of the ocean, representing fluidity and movement.

Weather Names

Storm - Symbolizing power and intensity, reminiscent of strong weather phenomena.

Raina - Derived from "rain," symbolizing refreshment and vitality.

Gale - Symbolizing strong winds, often associated with storms at sea.

Tempest - Evoking images of violent storms, symbolizing chaos and power.

Aurora - Named after the natural light display in the Earth's sky, symbolizing beauty and wonder.

Zephyr - Meaning a gentle, mild breeze, symbolizing tranquility and serenity.

Misty - Evoking images of fine droplets suspended in the air, symbolizing mystery and allure.

Thunder - Symbolizing the sound produced by lightning, often associated with storms.

Breeze - Representing a light, gentle wind, symbolizing calmness and relief.

Solstice - Referring to the longest or shortest day of the year, symbolizing change and transition.

Blaze - Evoking images of intense fire and heat, symbolizing passion and energy.

Dawn - Referring to the early morning light, symbolizing new beginnings and hope.

Cyclone - Symbolizing a rotating storm system, often associated with strong winds and rain.

Mistral - A strong, cold wind that blows from the northwest in southern France, symbolizing power and direction.

Haila - Derived from "hail," symbolizing resilience and strength in the face of adversity.

Skyler - Meaning "scholar" or "learned one," symbolizing knowledge and wisdom from observing the sky.

Sirocco - A hot, dry wind from northern Africa, symbolizing warmth and exoticism.

Monsoon - Referring to seasonal winds in South Asia, symbolizing change and renewal.

Sleet - Symbolizing a mixture of rain and snow, often associated with cold weather.

Cirrus - Named after wispy clouds high in the atmosphere, symbolizing delicacy and grace.

Haze - Referring to a fine suspension of moisture or dust in the air, symbolizing obscurity and mystery.

Nimbus - Referring to a cloud that produces precipitation, symbolizing fertility and abundance.

Frost - Symbolizing cold weather, often associated with ice and snow.

Celeste - Meaning "heavenly" or "of the sky," symbolizing transcendence and spirituality.

Aurora - Named after the natural light display in the Earth's sky, symbolizing beauty and wonder.

Literary Names

Dante - Inspired by Dante Alighieri, author of "The Divine Comedy," symbolizing exploration of the afterlife.

Ophelia - From Shakespeare's "Hamlet," symbolizing innocence and tragic beauty.

Holden - Inspired by J.D. Salinger's "The Catcher in the Rye," symbolizing rebellion and disillusionment.

Bronte - Inspired by the Bronte sisters, authors of classic novels like "Jane Eyre" and "Wuthering Heights," symbolizing literary prowess and creativity.

Atticus - From Harper Lee's "To Kill a Mockingbird," symbolizing moral integrity and wisdom.

Austen - Inspired by Jane Austen, author of classics like "Pride and Prejudice" and "Sense and Sensibility," symbolizing wit and romance.

Scout - From Harper Lee's "To Kill a Mockingbird," symbolizing curiosity and innocence.

Darcy - Inspired by Mr. Darcy from Jane Austen's "Pride and Prejudice," symbolizing aloofness and hidden depth.

Scarlett - Inspired by Scarlett O'Hara from Margaret Mitchell's "Gone with the Wind," symbolizing strength and resilience.

Heathcliff - From Emily Bronte's "Wuthering Heights," symbolizing passion and torment.

Gatsby - Inspired by F. Scott Fitzgerald's "The Great Gatsby," symbolizing the American Dream and decadence.

Cosette - From Victor Hugo's "Les Misérables," symbolizing innocence and redemption.

Arwen - Inspired by J.R.R. Tolkien's "The Lord of the Rings," symbolizing beauty and grace.

Rhett - Inspired by Rhett Butler from Margaret Mitchell's "Gone with the Wind," symbolizing charm and defiance.

Lisbeth - From Stieg Larsson's "The Girl with the Dragon Tattoo," symbolizing strength and resilience.

Frodo - From J.R.R. Tolkien's "The Lord of the Rings," symbolizing courage and perseverance.

Eowyn - Also from J.R.R. Tolkien's "The Lord of the Rings," symbolizing bravery and independence.

Jo - From Louisa May Alcott's "Little Women," symbolizing tomboyishness and ambition.

Lyra - From Philip Pullman's "His Dark Materials" trilogy, symbolizing curiosity and adventure.

Pippin - Also from J.R.R. Tolkien's "The Lord of the Rings," symbolizing loyalty and humor.

Viola - From Shakespeare's "Twelfth Night," symbolizing disguise and mistaken identity.

Aragorn - Also from J.R.R. Tolkien's "The Lord of the Rings," symbolizing nobility and leadership.

Hermione - From J.K. Rowling's "Harry Potter" series, symbolizing intelligence and loyalty.

Jay - Inspired by Jay Gatsby from F. Scott Fitzgerald's "The Great Gatsby," symbolizing ambition and idealism.

Scheherazade - From "One Thousand and One Nights," symbolizing storytelling and wit.

Harry Potter™ Characters

Harry - Inspired by the protagonist Harry Potter, symbolizing bravery and resilience.

Hermione - Symbolizing intelligence and loyalty, inspired by Hermione Granger.

Ron - Inspired by Harry's loyal friend Ron Weasley, symbolizing loyalty and humor.

Luna - Inspired by Luna Lovegood, symbolizing eccentricity and open-mindedness.

Neville - Inspired by Neville Longbottom, symbolizing bravery and growth.

Ginny - Inspired by Ginny Weasley, symbolizing strength and determination.

Draco - Inspired by Draco Malfoy, symbolizing ambition and cunning.

Sirius - Named after Sirius Black, symbolizing loyalty and courage.

Lily - Inspired by Lily Potter, symbolizing love and sacrifice.

Cedric - Inspired by Cedric Diggory, symbolizing fairness and kindness.

Bellatrix - Inspired by Bellatrix Lestrange, symbolizing madness and obsession.

Albus - Named after Albus Dumbledore, symbolizing wisdom and leadership.

Severus - Named after Severus Snape, symbolizing complexity and redemption.

Remus - Named after Remus Lupin, symbolizing resilience and acceptance.

Narcissa - Inspired by Narcissa Malfoy, symbolizing devotion and protection.

Minerva - Named after Minerva McGonagall, symbolizing strength and discipline.

Fleur - Inspired by Fleur Delacour, symbolizing beauty and grace.

Viktor - Inspired by Viktor Krum, symbolizing strength and determination.

Fred - Inspired by Fred Weasley, symbolizing humor and mischief.

George - Inspired by George Weasley, symbolizing loyalty and resilience.

Nymphadora - Inspired by Nymphadora Tonks, symbolizing uniqueness and adaptability.

Arthur - Named after Arthur Weasley, symbolizing kindness and curiosity.

Molly - Inspired by Molly Weasley, symbolizing warmth and maternal love.

Hagrid - Named after Rubeus Hagrid, symbolizing kindness and loyalty to creatures.

Cho - Inspired by Cho Chang, symbolizing sensitivity and loyalty.

Native American Names

Aiyana - Eternal blossom
Chaska - Star
Kiona - Brown hills
Takoda - Friend to everyone
Winona - Firstborn daughter
Aponi - Butterfly
Kachina - Spirit
Anoki - Actor
Ayita - First to dance
Nahimana - Mystical being
Enola - Solitary
Misu - Rippling water
Sequoia - Sparrow
Atsila - Fire
Kai - Willow tree
Odina - Mountain
Cheveyo - Spirit warrior
Takala - Corn tassel
Wicasa - Sage
Kitchi - Brave
Maka - Earth
Odakota - Friend
Nayati - Wrestler
Istas - Snow
Hotah - Warrior
Halona - Happy fortune
Kasa - Dressed in fur
Lenmana - Flute
Muna - Overflowing spring
Osage - Warrior
Orenda - Magic power
Powaqa - Witch
Shikoba - Feather
Tama - Thunderbolt

Una - Remember
Yoki - Rain
Zapotec - Ancient tribe
Elsu - Flying falcon
Hawiovi - Going away and returning
Isi - Deer
Jolon - Valley of the dead oaks
Catori - Spirit
Enola - Magnolia
Micco - Chief
Nita - Bear
Kangee - Raven
Opa - Owl
Lulu - Rabbit
Wapun - Dawn
Oota Dabun - Daystar
Taima - Thunder
Tadita - Running water
Tanis - Daughter of the wind
Tiva - Dance
Tuketu - Bear making noise
Adahy - Lives in the woods
Tala - Stalking wolf
Tallulah - Leaping water
Tayanita - Young beaver
Tiponi - Child of importance
Yansa - Buffalo
Yara - Seagull
Akecheta - Fighter

Aboriginal Names

Warragul - Eagle
Murrin - Honey
Yara - Seagull
Jarrah - Eucalyptus tree
Tarni - Wave
Jardi - Kangaroo
Nura - Country
Kiah - From the beautiful place
Kurrajong - Tree with gum
Miri - Star
Warrigal - Wild dog
Koora - Kangaroo
Mirrin - Kangaroo
Birra - Star
Dindi - Butterfly
Ginara - Emu
Mia - Home
Narla - Sun
Wandana - Friend
Billa - River
Djaran - Crow
Kalina - Love
Malu - Kangaroo
Pirra - Moon
Talia - Rain from heaven
Wambat - Wombat
Yindi - Sunlight
Dhara - Earth
Jarli - Cockatoo
Karri - Tree
Marni - Tomorrow
Nala - Rain
Oola - Moon

Maroi Names

Aroha - Love, compassion
Manaia - Guardian spirit
Hine - Girl, daughter
Tama - Boy, son
Hinemoa - Girl of great importance
Tane - Man, husband
Rangi - Sky, heavens
Hineamaru - Girl of peaceful disposition
Whetu - Star
Tangaroa - God of the sea
Marama - Moon
Hemi - James
Rongo - God of peace and cultivation
Kiri - Skin, bark
Tui - Bird known for its beautiful song
Mana - Prestige, authority
Kahu - Cloak, garment
Hiriwa - Silver
Pania - Mythical maiden who lived in the sea
Taika - Tiger
Tangi - Cry, weep
Awhina - Support, help
Tumatauenga - God of war
Maru - Shelter, protection
Anahera - Angel
Hauora - Health, well-being
Rua - Pit, hole
Tawhiri - God of weather, winds
Waiata - Song
Tangata - Person, human being
Moana - Ocean, sea
Hinekura - Girl of red earth
Maia - Brave, confident
Ruaumoko - God of earthquakes and volcanoes

Tapuwae - Footprint, track
Awa - River
Tane Mahuta - God of forests and birds
Ariki - Chief, leader
Hinewai - Girl of the water
Teina - Younger sibling
Whakapapa - Genealogy, ancestry
Kai - Food
Rongoa - Traditional medicine
Tangihanga - Funeral, mourning
Hira - Long, tall
Wairua - Spirit, soul
Whakairo - Carving, sculpture
Hinerau - Girl of the hills
Tawhirimatea - God of storms
Whenua - Land, earth
Tari - Office, bureau
Mataatua - Canoe of Maori mythology
Whakarongo - Listen, hear
Kowhai - Yellow flowering tree
Whakapono - Faith, belief
Mahi - Work, job
Moe - Sleep, rest
Hina - Silver, gray
Whakarere - Leave, depart
Manawa - Heart, center
Wairangi - Crazy, mad

Sami Names

Ailo - "Little wild one"
Inga - "Protected by Ing"
Mattis - "Gift of God"
Sága - "The seeing one"
Nils - "Champion"
Maja - "Pearl"
Aslak - "Godly support"
Siri - "Beautiful victory"
Isak - "Laughter"
Ida - "Work"
Aksel - "Father of peace"
Marja - "Beloved"
Ola - "Ancestor's relic"
Aila - "Diminutive of Helga, meaning 'holy, blessed'"
Mikkel - "Who is like God?"
Kaisa - "Pure"
Oskar - "Divine spear"
Sanna - "Lily"
Per - "Rock"
Greta - "Pearl"
Jovnna - "The grace of God"
Eira - "Snow"
Jon - "God is gracious"
Risten - "Baptism"
Niila - "Victorious people"
Siv - "Bride"
Alva - "Elf"
Nilsa - "Victory of the people"
Máret - "Pearl"
Johan - "God is gracious"
Maia - "Great"
Jaska - "Jasmine flower"
Sara - "Princess"
Trygve - "True, trustworthy"

Áddjá - "Father"
Beata - "Blessed"
Ante - "Priceless"
Silje - "Blind"
Eirik - "Forever strong"
Gull - "Gold"
Bente - "Blessed"
Elias - "The Lord is my God"
Maaren - "Rebellious"
Boazu - "Reindeer"
Astrid - "Beautiful, loved"
Markus - "Warlike"
Jussi - "God is gracious"
Malla - "Sea"
Torkel - "Thor's cauldron"
Egil - "Sword's edge"
Annika - "Grace"
Hilda - "Battle"
Kari - "Pure"
Sunniva - "Sun gift"
Åsa - "Godly strength"
Mihkkal - "Who is like God?"
Tuva - "Dove"
Arne - "Eagle"
Elin - "Torch of light"
Nanna - "Brave"
Njulla - "Aurora borealis"
Liv - "Life"
Rávnna - "Spear"
Gita - "Pearl"
Eline - "Torch of light"
Jona - "Dove"
Turi - "Rose"
Árja - "Eagle"
Biret - "Bright, famous"
Ánde - "Manly"

Inuit Names

Nanook - Polar bear
Aanaq - Wind
Sesi - Snow
Kalla - Thunder
Nuliajuk - Sea goddess
Aglukark - Hare
Nuka - Younger sibling
Anana - Mother
Uki - Survivor
Taqqiq - Moon
Aka - Elder sibling
Nootaikok - Wise owl
Suka - Fast
Pukak - Soapstone
Aningan - Great spirit
Inuk - Person
Siku - Ice
Taktuq - Caribou
Nuliaq - Moonlight
Iqaluk - Fish
Qimmiq - Dog
Panik - Daughter
Piqalujjaq - Snowflake
Nukilik - Beloved
Arnak - Woman
Quviasuktuq - Morning star
Sissiq - Baby seal
Taiga - Wolf
Kallik - Lightning
Qannik - Snowflake
Ula - Jewel
Nalik - Beautiful
Naja - Belonging to us
Suralik - Seagull

Pitsiulak - Woodpecker
Pikku - Child
Kallak - Whitefish
Qilaq - Sky
Taqtu - Frozen
Akinak - Dagger
Aatag - Dawn
Sila - Sky, universe
Illuliaq - Weather
Ivalu - House
Nuvvigaq - Snowy owl
Kavik - Wolverine
Panikpak - Butterfly
Niviarsiaq - She is a wise woman
Nalli - Sun
Anuraq - Snow bunting
Puuka - Seagull
Tulugaq - Raven
Akiak - Brave
Suluk - Feather
Imiq - Water
Kimmirut - Heel
Arnarulunnguaq - Little eagle
Piitaq - Beloved
Quviasuk - North Star
Nanurluk - Great bear
Anguta - Man's spirit
Qisuk - Fish
Agayu - Inland Eskimo
Kavivaar - Eskimo knife
Pukimna - Butterfly
Sialuk - Black
Kanaaq - Thunder
Ijiraq - Shape shifter
Silapaaq - Glow of the sun on the snow
Taqralik - Sky

Uvanga - Mine
Arnannuraq - Strong eagle
Pilu - Fairy
Tuktu - Caribou
Kanak - Earth
Tuluksak - Frost
Apik - Snowdrift
Kikila - Eskimo dance
Nilak - Celestial
Taranga - Moon
Qanuk - Star

Hawiian Names

Aka - Shadow
Alika - Noble, guardian
Alana - Awakening
Aleka - Defender of man
Alika - Defender of man
Anela - Angel
Elikapeka - Elizabeth
Elua - Second born
Haimi - Seeking knowledge
Hala - Fruit-bearing tree
Halia - Memorial, remembrance
Haukea - White snow
Hoku - Star
Hualani - Heavenly fruit
Hula - Dance
Ikaika - Strength
Ilima - Flower
Iolana - Soaring like a hawk
Kaipo - Sweetheart
Kalani - The heavens
Kalea - Bright, clear
Kalei - Beloved, adorned one
Kalena - Brightness, glow
Kalua - Second child
Kamea - The one and only
Kanoa - Free one
Kapua - Flower
Kaulana - Famous
Kawai - Water
Keahi - Flames, fire
Kealani - Chief
Keiki - Child
Kekoa - Brave one
Kiana - Divine, heavenly

Kiele - Fragrant blossom
Kiko - Second born
Kina - China
Koa - Warrior
Koali - Child of royal descent
Kokua - Help, assistance
Kona - Lady
Kuhina - Queen, regent
Lani - Sky, heavens
Lei - Garland of flowers
Liko - Bud
Lokelani - Small red rose
Luana - Content, happy
Mahina - Moon
Malia - Bitter, sea of bitterness
Mana - Spiritual power
Manuia - Happy, cheerful
Maile - Fragrant vine
Makana - Gift
Makani - Wind
Malu - Peace, protection
Malia - Calm, peaceful
Mano - Shark
Mele - Song
Miliani - Gentle caress
Nalani - The heavens
Noe - Mist, misty rain
Nalani - Calm skies
Nanea - Tranquil, leisurely
Nohea - Lovely, handsome
Olelo - Language, speech
Onaona - Sweet scent
Pualani - Heavenly flower
Pua - Flower
Puakea - White flower
Puanani - Beautiful flower

Uluwehi - Adorned with leaves
Umi - Sprout, growing
Wai - Water
Wahine - Woman
Wailana - Calm waters
Wainani - Beautiful water
Wakea - Sky father
Wahine - Girl, woman
Wehilani - Crown of heaven
Welina - Welcome
Waiola - Living water
Waipuna - Spring water
Wahine - Female, woman
Wailua - Two waters
Walina - The heavens
Waihee - Fresh water
Waimanu - Bird-like water
Wainui - Big water
Waiola - Water of life
Waipele - Explosive water
Wahine - Girl, lady
Weuweu - Green mist
Waiola - Shimmering water
Waikiki - Spouting water
Waikea - Expansive water
Wailoa - Long water
Waimalu - Peaceful water
Waihua - Refreshing water
Wailana - Gentle water
Waika - Strong water

Military Names

Victor - Conqueror, winner
Maximus - Greatest
Valentina - Strong, brave
Felix - Lucky, fortunate
Athena - Goddess of wisdom and war
Conrad - Bold counsel
Victoria - Victory
Roland - Famous land
Bianca - White, pure
Theodore - Gift of God
Cassandra - Helper of mankind
Gunner - Soldier who operates a gun
Isadora - Gift of Isis (ancient Egyptian goddess of fertility and motherhood)
Lysander - Liberator
Astrid - Divine strength
Magnus - Great, large
Andromeda - Ruler of men
Garrison - Guarded town
Callista - Most beautiful
Ajax - Eagle
Mila - Gracious, dear
Evander - Good man
Cadence - Rhythmic flow
Mars - Roman god of war
Juno - Queen of the gods (Roman mythology)
Damon - To tame, subdue
Nikita - Victorious
Thalia - Flourishing, blooming
Leonidas - Lion-like
Aurora - Goddess of dawn
Ethan - Strong, firm
Xenia - Hospitality, friendliness
Evita - Living, lively

Marcus - Warlike
Freya - Norse goddess of love and war
Quentin - Fifth
Thea - Goddess, divine
Caspian - From the Caspian Sea region
Ares - Greek god of war
Ariadne - Most holy
Axel - Father of peace
Liberty - Freedom, independence
Thaddeus - Courageous heart
Gaia - Earth goddess
Griffin - Strong lord
Nyx - Goddess of the night
Ranger - Warrior who operates in rough terrain

Slavic Names

Aleksander - Defender of mankind
Natalia - Born on Christmas Day
Maksim - Greatest
Katarina - Pure
Ivan - God is gracious
Milena - Gracious, dear
Dmitri - Earth-lover
Yelena - Bright, shining light
Anton - Priceless
Luka - Light
Marina - From the sea
Bogdan - Given by God
Sofiya - Wisdom
Andrei - Brave, manly
Zoya - Life
Pavel - Small
Vera - Faith
Nikita - Unconquered
Svetlana - Light
Roman - Citizen of Rome
Anastasia - Resurrection
Sergei - Servant
Yekaterina - Pure
Vladislav - Rule with glory
Anna - Gracious
Mikhail - Who is like God?
Irina - Peace
Stanislav - Glorious government
Elena - Shining light
Viktor - Conqueror
Ksenia - Hospitable
Igor - Warrior
Varvara - Foreign woman
Yaroslav - Bright fame

Tatyana - Fairy queen
Yuri - Farmer
Alina - Bright, beautiful
Artyom - Safe, sound
Galina - Calm, tranquil
Danil - God is my judge
Polina - Small
Dmitri - Earth-lover
Natalya - Born on Christmas Day
Ilya - Jehovah is God
Yuliya - Youthful
Semyon - God has heard
Anastasiya - Resurrection
Nikita - Unconquered
Veronika - True image
Fyodor - Gift of God
Zinaida - Life of Zeus
Vasily - King
Mila - Gracious, dear
Yevgeny - Well-born
Raisa - Easy, light-hearted
Stepan - Crown
Valentina - Strong, healthy
Mariya - Bitter
Alexei - Defender
Yelizaveta - God is my oath
Miroslav - Peaceful glory
Yaroslava - Bright and glorious
Vadim - Ruler, judge
Yelena - Bright, shining light
Kira - Ladylike
Boris - Battle glory
Miloslav - Gracious glory
Zoya - Life
Antonina - Priceless
Konstantin - Steadfast

Yelizaveta - God is my oath
Lev - Lion
Lyudmila - Loved by the people
Grigori - Vigilant
Irina - Peace
Stanislav - Glorious government
Vera - Faith
Aleksandra - Defender of mankind
Radoslav - Happy glory
Anastasiya - Resurrection
Pavel - Small
Yaroslav - Bright fame
Antonia - Priceless
Vladimir - Rule with greatness
Oksana - Praise be to God
Bogdana - Given by God
Leonid - Lion
Milena - Gracious, dear
Sofiya - Wisdom
Anatoly - Sunrise
Yekaterina - Pure
Raisa - Easy, light-hearted
Igor - Warrior
Nina - Grace
Timofei - One who honors God
Larisa - Cheerful
Yulia - Youthful
Vadim - Ruler, judge
Elena - Shining light
Aleksandr - Defender of mankind

Saxon Names

Aethelstan - Noble stone
Wulfhere - Wolf army
Eadric - Wealthy ruler
Leofwine - Beloved friend
Aelfric - Elf ruler
Godwin - God friend
Leofsige - Beloved victory
Aethelflaed - Noble beauty
Eadburg - Wealthy fortress
Leofric - Beloved ruler
Beornheard - Brave and strong
Hrothgar - Famous spear
Wulfstan - Wolf stone
Ealdgyth - Old battle
Aelfweard - Elf guardian
Godiva - God gift
Leofgyth - Beloved war
Aethelred - Noble counsel
Eadgyth - Wealthy battle
Edric - Wealthy ruler
Aethelwine - Noble friend
Wulfric - Wolf power
Eadwulf - Wealthy wolf
Aelfgar - Elf spear
Godric - God ruler
Leofa - Dear, beloved
Aethelwyn - Noble joy
Eadmund - Wealthy protector
Aelfflaed - Elf beauty
Wulfgar - Wolf spear
Eadred - Wealthy counsel

Celtic Names

Aiden - Fiery one
Bran - Raven
Ciaran - Dark one
Declan - Full of goodness
Eavan - Fair or beautiful
Fionn - Fair or white
Grania - Love
Eilidh - Sun or radiant one
Lachlan - Land of lakes
Maeve - Intoxicating
Niamh - Bright or radiant
Oran - Pale green
Rhys - Enthusiasm
Sinead - God is gracious
Ailbhe - White or fair
Bevan - Son of Evan
Daire - Oak tree
Eira - Snow
Finley - Fair-haired hero
Gwendolyn - White ring
Isolde - Beautiful
Kian - Ancient or enduring
Mairead - Pearl
Niall - Champion
Oisin - Little deer
Rhiannon - Great queen
Sorcha - Bright or radiant
Tadhg - Poet or philosopher
Aisling - Dream or vision
Blaine - Thin or slender
Darragh - Oak tree
Enya - Kernel or grain
Fiona - Fair or white
Gareth - Gentle or modest

Imogen - Maiden
Keira - Dark or black
Lir - Song of the sea
Malachy - Servant of Saint Maelruain
Nuala - White shoulder
Owen - Young warrior
Riona - Queenly
Siobhan - God is gracious
Taliesin - Shining brow
Una - Lamb
Aine - Radiance or brightness
Brigid - Exalted one
Eamon - Wealthy guardian
Giselle - Pledge or hostage
Idris - Fiery or impulsive
Lorna - Sorrowful

Ancient Welsh Names

Aneirin - Noble
Branwen - Beautiful raven
Caradog - Beloved friend
Dylan - Sea
Eleri - Bitter or sacred
Glyn - Valley
Heulwen - Sunshine
Idris - Fiery or impulsive
Llewelyn - Lion-like
Morwen - Waves of the sea
Rhodri - Wheel king
Seren - Star
Taliesin - Shining brow
Aderyn - Bird
Bronwen - Fair breast
Cai - Rejoice
Dyfan - Beloved
Eira - Snow
Gwilym - Resolute protector
Islwyn - Below the grove
Llinos - Flaxen-haired
Myfanwy - My fine one
Rhian - Maiden
Tegan - Toy or darling
Alun - Harmony
Cadfael - Battle prince
Deryn - Bird
Eirian - Silver
Gethin - Dark-skinned
Ianto - God is gracious
Lleu - Light
Nerys - Lady
Rhiannon - Great queen
Tegwen - Beautiful

Angharad - Much loved
Caryl - Beloved
Dilys - Genuine
Eluned - Image or idol
Gwennan - Fair or blessed
Iestyn - Righteous
Llew - Lion
Nest - Pure
Rhys - Enthusiasm
Tecwyn - Beautiful prince
Arwel - High noble
Catrin - Pure
Dafydd - Beloved
Eleri - Bitter or sacred
Gwenllian - White, fair or blessed
Idris - Fiery or impulsive

Persian Names

Amir - Prince, ruler
Ava - Voice, sound
Cyrus - Sun
Leyla - Night, dark beauty
Farid - Unique, precious
Yasmin - Jasmine flower
Ramin - Enlightened, wise
Soraya - Star
Kian - King, royal
Shadi - Joyful, happy
Darya - Sea
Arman - Desire, hope
Parisa - Like a fairy, graceful
Roshan - Bright, shining
Neda - Voice, call
Farshad - Happiness, joy
Laleh - Tulip flower
Reza - Contentment, satisfaction
Nika - Good, victory
Sahar - Dawn, morning
Aria - Noble, honorable
Bijan - Heroic, brave
Sanaz - Graceful, elegant
Soroush - Messenger, angel
Samira - Pleasant companion
Bijan - Heroic, brave
Behnam - Reputable, honorable
Afsaneh - Story, legend
Mehran - Kind, generous
Shahrzad - City dweller
Sina - Spear, warrior
Parviz - Victorious, triumphant
Niloufar - Lotus flower
Kiana - Royal, regal

Arash - Bright, radiant
Nargis - Narcissus flower
Armin - Protector, defender
Mahin - Moon-like
Ashkan - Good natured, cheerful
Shirin - Sweet, pleasant
Bardia - Prince, nobleman
Sahar - Awakening, dawn
Farhad - Happiness, joy
Nasrin - Wild rose
Kourosh - Sun-like, radiant
Shiraz - Famous wine, city in Iran
Mitra - Friend, ally
Ardeshir - Righteous, holy
Zara - Princess, flower
Mehrdad - Gift of love

Lucky Names

Asher - Happy and blessed
Felicity - Good fortune and happiness
Bennett - Blessed
Evangeline - Bringer of good news
Chance - Luck or fortune
Aurora - Dawn, symbolizing new beginnings
Felix - Lucky, fortunate
Beatrice - Bringer of joy and blessings
Benedict - Blessed
Esme - Esteemed or beloved, bringing good luck
Nadira - Rare and precious, symbolizing good fortune
Edmund - Prosperous protector
Mira - Prosperous and peaceful
Ashlyn - Dream or vision, bringing luck
Zane - Gift from God, symbolizing luck
Lucy - Light, bringing brightness and luck
Hugo - Intelligent and wise, bringing good fortune
Nadia - Hope or new beginnings
Asha - Hope or wish, symbolizing luck
Naomi - Pleasant, bringing happiness and good fortune
Kiara - Bright, bringing luck and prosperity

Food Based Names

Olive - Symbol of peace and fruitfulness
Basil - Royal or kingly
Sage - Wise or knowledgeable
Ginger - Energetic or lively
Rosemary - Dew of the sea; symbol of remembrance
Pepper - Fiery or spicy
Cayenne - Named after the hot pepper variety
Saffron - Precious spice; symbol of wealth and prosperity
Thyme - Courageous or strong-willed
Clementine - Gentle or merciful
Clement - Derived from Clementine; gentle or merciful
Cinnamon - Sweet and spicy; symbol of warmth and comfort
Coco - Diminutive form of Cocoa; relating to chocolate
Honey - Sweetness and nourishment
Berry - Small fruit; symbol of growth and fertility
Cherry - Symbol of love and passion
Cocoa - Derived from the cacao bean; associated with chocolate
Colby - Meaning uncertain; often associated with the cheese variety
Kale - Named after the leafy green vegetable
Lemon - Sour and refreshing; symbol of vitality
Lychee - Sweet and exotic fruit
Mango - Tropical fruit; symbol of abundance and fertility
Paprika - Named after the spice derived from peppers
Peach - Sweet and juicy fruit; symbol of longevity and happiness
Peanut - Small and nutritious; symbol of humility and simplicity
Pistachio - Nutritious and flavorful nut
Plum - Sweet and succulent fruit
Pumpkin - Symbol of harvest and abundance; associated with autumn

Tamarind - Sweet and tangy fruit
Tapioca - Derived from the starch extracted from cassava roots
Vanilla - Sweet and fragrant spice

Gem Names

Pearl - Precious gem formed within the shell of an oyster; symbolizes purity and innocence.

Ruby - Precious gemstone; symbolizes love, passion, and vitality.

Emerald - Precious gemstone; symbolizes growth, renewal, and prosperity.

Sapphire - Precious gemstone; symbolizes wisdom, truth, and intuition.

Topaz - Gemstone; symbolizes strength, healing, and enlightenment.

Amber - Fossilized tree resin; symbolizes warmth, energy, and protection.

Onyx - Gemstone; symbolizes strength, resilience, and self-control.

Garnet - Gemstone; symbolizes love, devotion, and regeneration.

Opal - Precious gemstone; symbolizes creativity, inspiration, and imagination.

Coral - Marine invertebrate; symbolizes protection, transformation, and peace.

Crystal - Clear mineral; symbolizes clarity, harmony, and spiritual growth.

Quartz - Mineral; symbolizes energy, clarity, and amplification.

Jade - Precious mineral; symbolizes purity, wisdom, and harmony.

Agate - Gemstone; symbolizes balance, stability, and protection.

Amethyst - Gemstone; symbolizes peace, tranquility, and spiritual awareness.

Beryl - Mineral; symbolizes purity, strength, and healing.

Citrine - Gemstone; symbolizes abundance, success, and prosperity.

Diamond - Precious gemstone; symbolizes purity, strength, and everlasting love.

Fluorite - Mineral; symbolizes clarity, focus, and mental enhancement.

Lapis - Gemstone; symbolizes truth, wisdom, and self-expression.

Malachite - Mineral; symbolizes transformation, protection, and healing.

Peridot - Gemstone; symbolizes happiness, prosperity, and good fortune.

Pyrite - Mineral; symbolizes abundance, protection, and vitality.

Tourmaline - Gemstone; symbolizes balance, compassion, and inspiration.

Celestite - Mineral; symbolizes peace, harmony, and divine guidance.

Hematite - Mineral; symbolizes grounding, protection, and strength.

Moonstone - Gemstone; symbolizes intuition, dreams, and emotional balance.

Obsidian - Volcanic glass; symbolizes protection, strength, and truth.

Rhodochrosite - Gemstone; symbolizes love, compassion, and self-discovery.

Serpentine - Mineral; symbolizes transformation, healing, and renewal.

Turquoise - Gemstone; symbolizes protection, communication, and spiritual expansion.

Amazonite - Gemstone; symbolizes balance, harmony, and personal truth.

Kunzite - Gemstone; symbolizes love, emotional healing, and peace.

Larimar - Gemstone; symbolizes tranquility, serenity, and inner wisdom.

Azurite - Mineral; symbolizes intuition, insight, and spiritual growth.

Rhodonite - Gemstone; symbolizes compassion, forgiveness, and emotional healing.

Artist Names

Frida Kahlo - Mexican artist known for her self-portraits that explore themes of identity, gender, and the human experience, often incorporating elements of Mexican culture and symbolism.

Wassily Kandinsky - Russian painter and art theorist credited with painting one of the first purely abstract works, "Composition IV," and a prominent figure in the development of abstract art.

Henri de Toulouse-Lautrec - French Post-Impressionist painter known for his depictions of Parisian nightlife, particularly cabaret and theater scenes.

Joan Miró - Spanish Surrealist artist known for his biomorphic forms, playful use of color, and childlike imagery, as seen in works like "The Tilled Field" and "The Smile of the Flamboyant Wings."

Gustav Klimt - Austrian Symbolist painter known for his decorative style, ornate patterns, and sensual portraits, including "The Kiss" and "Portrait of Adele Bloch-Bauer I."

Rene Magritte - Belgian Surrealist artist known for his thought-provoking and enigmatic paintings that challenge the viewer's perception of reality, such as "The Son of Man" and "The Treachery of Images."

Paul Cézanne - French Post-Impressionist painter known for his innovative approach to form and color, particularly in his landscapes and still lifes, laying the groundwork for Cubism and modern art.

Mary Cassatt - American Impressionist painter known for her intimate portraits of mothers and children, capturing tender moments of domestic life with sensitivity and grace.

Sports Stars Names

Michael Jordan (Basketball): Widely regarded as the greatest basketball player of all time, Jordan won six NBA championships with the Chicago Bulls and earned five regular-season MVP awards. His extraordinary skills, competitiveness, and clutch performances have left an indelible mark on the sport.

Serena Williams (Tennis): With 23 Grand Slam singles titles, Serena Williams is one of the most dominant and successful tennis players in history. Her powerful serve, athleticism, and mental fortitude have made her a legend in the sport.

Usain Bolt (Track and Field): Known as the fastest man in the world, Usain Bolt has won eight Olympic gold medals and holds the world records in both the 100 meters and 200 meters. His unparalleled speed and charisma have made him a global icon.

Pelé (Soccer): Regarded as one of the greatest soccer players of all time, Pelé won three FIFA World Cups with the Brazilian national team and scored over 1,000 career goals. His exceptional skill, vision, and goal-scoring ability have solidified his legacy in the sport.

Muhammad Ali (Boxing): A three-time heavyweight champion and Olympic gold medalist, Muhammad Ali is considered one of the most significant and celebrated athletes in history. Known for his charisma, poetic trash talk, and boxing prowess, Ali transcended the sport to become a global icon of courage and social activism.

Roger Federer (Tennis): With 20 Grand Slam singles titles, Roger Federer is widely regarded as one of the greatest tennis players of all time. His elegant playing style, versatility, and longevity have earned him admiration from fans and fellow athletes alike.

Tom Brady (American Football): Considered by many as the greatest quarterback in NFL history, Tom Brady has won seven Super Bowl championships, the most by any player in NFL history. His leadership, clutch performances, and ability to excel under pressure have made him a football legend.

Lionel Messi (Soccer): Known for his exceptional dribbling skills, vision, and goal-scoring ability, Lionel Messi is widely regarded as one of the greatest soccer players of all time. With numerous individual awards and records, Messi has left an indelible mark on the sport.

Michael Phelps (Swimming): The most decorated Olympian of all time, Michael Phelps has won 23 Olympic gold medals and set numerous world records in swimming. His unparalleled dominance in the pool and dedication to his craft have solidified his status as a swimming legend.

Jackie Joyner-Kersee (Track and Field): Regarded as one of the greatest female athletes of all time, Jackie Joyner-Kersee won three Olympic gold medals and one silver medal in the heptathlon and long jump. Her versatility, athleticism, and longevity have earned her widespread acclaim in track and field.

Saints Names

Saint Francis of Assisi: Known for his love of nature and animals, Saint Francis is the patron saint of animals and the environment. He founded the Franciscan Order, embracing a life of poverty, simplicity, and service to the poor.

Saint Teresa of Calcutta (Mother Teresa): Renowned for her work among the poor and sick in Kolkata (Calcutta), India, Mother Teresa dedicated her life to serving the most marginalized and vulnerable members of society. She founded the Missionaries of Charity, which operates hospices, homes for the disabled, and orphanages worldwide.

Saint Patrick: The patron saint of Ireland, Saint Patrick is credited with bringing Christianity to Ireland. He is celebrated on March 17th, the date of his death, with the holiday of St. Patrick's Day, which has become a cultural celebration of Irish heritage around the world.

Saint Joan of Arc: Known as the Maid of Orleans, Saint Joan of Arc was a French peasant girl who claimed to have received visions from saints urging her to support Charles VII and help drive the English from France during the Hundred Years' War. She was later captured, tried for heresy, and burned at the stake.

Saint Nicholas: Also known as Santa Claus, Saint Nicholas was a 4th-century Christian bishop in Myra, Asia Minor (modern-day Turkey). He was known for his generosity and secret gift-giving, which inspired the tradition of Santa Claus.

Saint Augustine of Hippo: A prolific writer and theologian, Saint Augustine played a significant role in the development of Christian theology. His works, such as "Confessions" and "City of God," have had a lasting influence on Christian thought.

Saint Theresa of Lisieux (The Little Flower): A French Carmelite nun, Saint Theresa is known for her autobiography, "Story of a Soul," which describes her "little way" of spiritual childhood and devotion to God in everyday life. She is revered for her simplicity, humility, and deep faith.

Saint Anthony of Padua: A Portuguese Franciscan friar, Saint Anthony is revered as the patron saint of lost things and the poor. He is also known for his powerful preaching and miracles, as well as his devotion to the Eucharist.

Saint Catherine of Siena: A mystic, theologian, and Doctor of the Church, Saint Catherine played a key role in the Avignon Papacy and Great Schism of the Catholic Church in the 14th century. She is known for her spiritual writings and advocacy for the poor and marginalized.

Saint Benedict of Nursia: The founder of Western Christian monasticism, Saint Benedict is best known for his Rule of Saint Benedict, a guide for communal living and prayer in monastic communities. His rule emphasizes humility, obedience, and balance in daily life.

Political Leaders Names

Nelson Mandela: As the first black president of South Africa, Mandela was a symbol of reconciliation and forgiveness following the end of apartheid. He promoted peace, equality, and social justice, and his leadership helped unite a divided nation.

Mahatma Gandhi: Known for his philosophy of nonviolent resistance, Gandhi led India to independence from British rule through peaceful protests and civil disobedience. His principles of truth, ahimsa (nonviolence), and satyagraha (civil disobedience) inspired movements for civil rights and freedom around the world.

Abraham Lincoln: As the 16th President of the United States, Lincoln led the country through one of its most challenging periods, the Civil War. He is remembered for his leadership, integrity, and commitment to preserving the Union and abolishing slavery.

Martin Luther King Jr.: A prominent leader in the American civil rights movement, King advocated for racial equality and justice through nonviolent resistance. His powerful speeches and peaceful protests helped bring about significant changes in American society, including the Civil Rights Act of 1964 and the Voting Rights Act of 1965.

Mother Teresa: Renowned for her compassion and selfless service to the poor and sick, Mother Teresa dedicated her life to caring for the most marginalized members of society. Her humanitarian work with the Missionaries of Charity earned her widespread admiration and respect.

Queen Elizabeth II: As the longest-reigning monarch in British history, Queen Elizabeth II has provided stability and continuity to the United Kingdom and the Commonwealth. Her sense of duty, dedication, and commitment to public service have earned her widespread affection and respect.

Dalai Lama: The spiritual leader of Tibetan Buddhism, the Dalai Lama is revered for his teachings on compassion, tolerance, and inner peace. His efforts to promote dialogue, nonviolence, and human rights have made him a beloved figure worldwide.

Ellen Johnson Sirleaf: The first female president of Liberia and the first elected female head of state in Africa, Sirleaf led her country through a period of recovery and reconstruction following years of civil war. Known as the "Iron Lady," she is celebrated for her leadership, resilience, and commitment to democracy.

Jacinda Ardern: As the Prime Minister of New Zealand, Ardern has gained international acclaim for her compassionate and inclusive leadership style. She has shown empathy and strength in times of crisis, including her response to the Christchurch mosque shootings and the COVID-19 pandemic.

Aung San Suu Kyi: A Nobel Peace Prize laureate and pro-democracy leader in Myanmar, Suu Kyi has long been admired for her courage and determination in the face of adversity. Despite facing years of house arrest and persecution, she has remained committed to the fight for democracy and human rights in her country.

Philosphers Names

Socrates: An ancient Greek philosopher known for his Socratic method of questioning and his emphasis on self-examination and critical thinking. Socrates' teachings focused on ethics, virtue, and the pursuit of knowledge, and he is considered one of the founders of Western philosophy.

Plato: A student of Socrates and the teacher of Aristotle, Plato founded the Academy in Athens, one of the earliest institutions of higher learning in the Western world. His dialogues explore a wide range of philosophical topics, including ethics, politics, metaphysics, and epistemology. Plato's theory of forms and his allegory of the cave are among his most influential ideas.

Aristotle: A towering figure in ancient Greek philosophy, Aristotle made significant contributions to logic, metaphysics, ethics, politics, and natural sciences. He is known for his empirical approach to knowledge and his systematic examination of the natural world. Aristotle's works, including "Nicomachean Ethics" and "Politics," continue to be studied and debated to this day.

Immanuel Kant: A central figure in modern philosophy, Kant sought to reconcile rationalism and empiricism while revolutionizing metaphysics, epistemology, and ethics. His "Critique of Pure Reason" and "Groundwork of the Metaphysics of Morals" are foundational texts in Western philosophy. Kant's moral philosophy, based on the categorical imperative, remains influential in contemporary ethical theory.

David Hume: A Scottish philosopher and empiricist, Hume challenged traditional notions of causality, induction, and personal identity. His works, including "A Treatise of Human Nature" and "Dialogues Concerning Natural Religion," had a profound impact on subsequent philosophical thought, particularly in the areas of skepticism and empiricism.

Rene Descartes: Often regarded as the father of modern philosophy, Descartes was a French philosopher, mathematician, and scientist. He is best known for his statement "Cogito, ergo sum" ("I think, therefore I am"), which epitomizes his method of doubt and his quest for certainty in knowledge. Descartes' dualism of mind and body and his contributions to analytical geometry are also noteworthy.

Friedrich Nietzsche: A German philosopher known for his critiques of religion, morality, and modernity, Nietzsche challenged conventional values and championed individualism, creativity, and the will to power. His works, including "Thus Spoke Zarathustra" and "Beyond Good and Evil," explore themes of nihilism, eternal recurrence, and the Ubermensch (overman).

John Stuart Mill: A British philosopher and economist, Mill was a leading advocate of utilitarianism, the ethical theory that actions are right to the extent that they promote happiness or pleasure and wrong to the extent that they produce pain or suffering. His works, including "On Liberty" and "Utilitarianism," continue to influence debates about freedom, justice, and morality.

Jean-Paul Sartre: A French existentialist philosopher and novelist, Sartre is known for his existentialist views on freedom, choice, and the absurdity of human existence. His concept of "existence precedes essence" emphasizes the individual's responsibility for creating meaning in a world devoid of inherent purpose. Sartre's works, such as "Being and Nothingness" and "No Exit," explore themes of existential angst and authenticity.

Confucius: An ancient Chinese philosopher and teacher, Confucius emphasized the importance of moral cultivation, social harmony, and filial piety. His teachings, compiled in the "Analects," advocate for ethical leadership, virtuous conduct, and the cultivation of benevolent relationships.

Floral Names

Rose: Symbolizes love, beauty, and passion.

Lily: Represents purity, innocence, and fertility.

Daisy: Signifies purity, innocence, and new beginnings.

Violet: Symbolizes modesty, faithfulness, and virtue.

Jasmine: Represents grace, elegance, and sensuality.

Poppy: Symbolizes remembrance, consolation, and eternal sleep.

Lavender: Represents calmness, tranquility, and relaxation.

Dahlia: Signifies inner strength, elegance, and dignity.

Iris: Symbolizes wisdom, courage, and faith.

Magnolia: Represents beauty, dignity, and nobility.

Peony: Signifies prosperity, good fortune, and romance.

Hyacinth: Symbolizes sincerity, forgiveness, and playfulness.

Camellia: Represents admiration, perfection, and longing.

Zinnia: Signifies endurance, remembrance, and friendship.

Chrysanthemum: Symbolizes loyalty, longevity, and joy.

Freesia: Represents friendship, innocence, and thoughtfulness.

Tulip: Signifies perfect love, passion, and elegance.

Orchid: Symbolizes luxury, beauty, and strength.

Hydrangea: Represents gratitude, understanding, and heartfelt emotions.

Sunflower: Signifies happiness, adoration, and vitality.

Azalea: Symbolizes femininity, passion, and balance.

Gardenia: Represents purity, love, and refinement.

Lilac: Signifies youthful innocence, confidence, and memories.

Carnation: Symbolizes love, fascination, and admiration.

Amaryllis: Represents pride, determination, and radiant beauty.

Anemone: Signifies anticipation, protection, and fragility.

Bluebell: Symbolizes humility, gratitude, and everlasting love.

Daffodil: Signifies rebirth, new beginnings, and hope.

Hibiscus: Symbolizes beauty, passion, and delicate charm.

Foxglove: Represents healing, protection, and magical energy.

Marigold: Signifies joy, success, and vibrant energy.

Primrose: Symbolizes youth, eternal love, and admiration.

Snowdrop: Signifies hope, purity, and renewal.

Verbena: Symbolizes enchantment, creativity, and healing.

Yarrow: Represents courage, healing, and protection..

Calla Lily: Symbolizes elegance, purity, and resurrection.

Pansy: Represents thoughtfulness, loyalty, and remembrance.

Quince: Signifies prosperity, love, and protection.

Tiger Lily: Signifies pride, confidence, and wealth.

Wisteria: Symbolizes long-life, beauty, and love.

Yarrow: Represents healing, protection, and courage.

Zephyranthes (Rain Lily): Signifies beauty, freshness, and renewal.

Printed in Great Britain
by Amazon